Editor

Pedro Weisleder

Nationwide Children's Hospital, USA
& The Ohio State University, USA

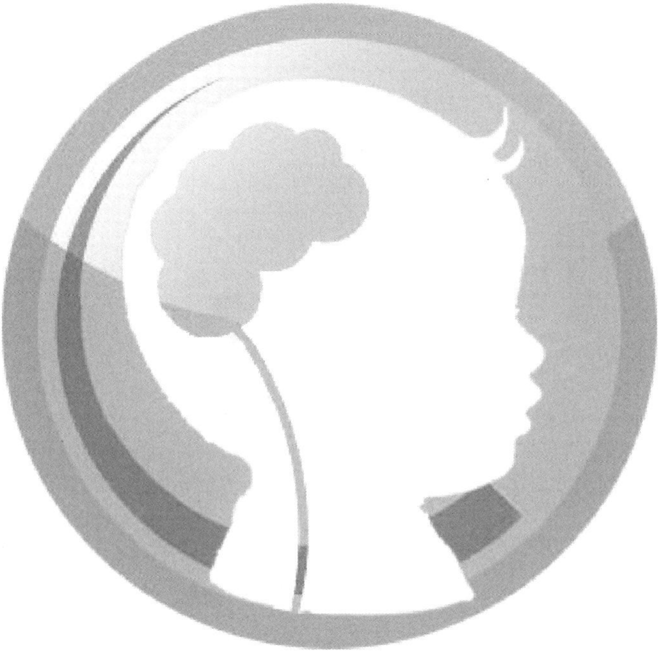

MANUAL OF PEDIATRIC NEUROLOGY

World Scientific

NEW JERSEY • LONDON • SINGAPORE • BEIJING • SHANGHAI • HONG KONG • TAIPEI • CHENNAI

Published by

World Scientific Publishing Co. Pte. Ltd.
5 Toh Tuck Link, Singapore 596224
USA office: 27 Warren Street, Suite 401-402, Hackensack, NJ 07601
UK office: 57 Shelton Street, Covent Garden, London WC2H 9HE

British Library Cataloguing-in-Publication Data
A catalogue record for this book is available from the British Library.

MANUAL OF PEDIATRIC NEUROLOGY

ISBN 978-981-4324-19-9

Typeset by Stallion Press
Email: enquiries@stallionpress.com

Printed in Singapore by Mainland Press Pte Ltd.

I dedicate this book to Deb, my wife, for her companionship and unwavering confidence which have made this and other endeavors possible.

To my parents, Flora and Moisés, for their love and support.

PREFACE

Editor: Pedro Weisleder, M.D., Ph.D.

Child neurology is a discipline that is experiencing very rapid change. New genetic and imaging tests are affording us the possibility to identify conditions that in the past were only diagnosed at autopsy. And yet, the case history and physical exam continue to be the cornerstones of the neurological evaluation. This book is for people who want to learn the foundations of child neurology. To that end, the authors and I designed this manual to be an easy to read and easy to access text based on clinical scenarios. The emphasis is on signs and symptoms, diagnostic tests as needed, and practical advice for treatment. By glancing at the chapters' titles, the reader can ascertain which topics we considered to be of particular importance. Some authors addressed mainstream and commonly encountered topics such as the management of seizures, headaches, and tic disorders. Others reviewed current knowledge on clinical issues that call for increasing awareness on the part of the pediatric neurologist such as idiopathic intracranial hypertension, neonatal neurology, and the management of stroke in children. The book's matter also covers topics tangentially related to neurology such as syncope, vetricluo-peritoneal shunt failure, and central nervous system infections. Finally, one chapter is devoted to the care of child neurology patients at the end of life.

As the editor, my primary goal was to produce a collection of chapters that addresses frequently encountered scenarios in all clinical settings. In addition, I was pleased to have been able to provide a forum not only for seasoned and well-established authors, but also for up-and-coming child neurologists. To end, I wish to thank my colleagues for their contributions. I recognize they are all busy individuals whose time for discretionary projects such as this book is limited and precious. Their efforts are greatly appreciated.

CONTENTS

CONTRIBUTORS

Shawn Aylward, M.D.
Division of Neurology
Nationwide Children's Hospital and The Ohio State University
Columbus, Ohio, USA

Dennis Cunningham, M.D.
Division of Infectious Diseases
Nationwide Children's Hospital and The Ohio State University
Columbus, Ohio, USA

Emily de los Reyes, M.D.
Division of Neurology
Nationwide Children's Hospital and The Ohio State University
Columbus, Ohio, USA

Emile El-Shammaa, M.D.
Division of Emergency Medicine
Nationwide Children's Hospital and The Ohio State University
Columbus, Ohio, USA

Gloria Galloway, M.D.
Division of Neurology
Nationwide Children's Hospital and The Ohio State University
Columbus, Ohio, USA

Timothy M. Hoffman, M.D.
Division of Cardiology
Nationwide Children's Hospital and The Ohio State University
Columbus, Ohio, USA

Monica Islam, M.D.
Division of Neurology
Nationwide Children's Hospital and The Ohio State University
Columbus, Ohio, USA

Eric M. Jackson, M.D.
Division of Neurosurgery
Nationwide Children's Hospital and The Ohio State University
Columbus, Ohio, USA

Latif Khuhro, M.D.
Division of Neurology
Nationwide Children's Hospital and The Ohio State University
Columbus, Ohio, USA

Lenora Lehwald, M.D.
Division of Neurology
Nationwide Children's Hospital and The Ohio State University
Columbus, Ohio, USA

Warren D. Lo, M.D.
Division of Neurology
Nationwide Children's Hospital and The Ohio State University
Columbus, Ohio, USA

Ann Pakalnis, M.D.
Division of Neurology
Nationwide Children's Hospital and The Ohio State University
Columbus, Ohio, USA

Anup Patel, M.D.
Division of Neurology
Nationwide Children's Hospital and The Ohio State University
Columbus, Ohio, USA

Corey Raffel, M.D., Ph.D.
Department of Neurosurgery
The Ohio State University
Columbus, Ohio, USA

E. Steve Roach, M.D.
Division of Neurology
Nationwide Children's Hospital and The Ohio State University
Columbus, Ohio, USA

Kimberly Scansen, M.D.
Division of Emergency Medicine
Nationwide Children's Hospital and The Ohio State University
Columbus, Ohio, USA

Laurel Slaughter, M.D.
Division of Neurology
Nationwide Children's Hospital and The Ohio State University
Columbus, Ohio, USA

Rachel Smitek, M.D.
Division of Emergency Medicine
Nationwide Children's Hospital and The Ohio State University
Columbus, Ohio, USA

Jack R. Stines, M.D.
Division of Cardiology
Nationwide Children's Hospital and The Ohio State University
Columbus, Ohio, USA

Shane F. Tsai, M.D.
Division of Cardiology
Nationwide Children's Hospital and The Ohio State University
Columbus, Ohio, USA

Chang-Yong Tsao, M.D.
Division of Neurology
Nationwide Children's Hospital and The Ohio State University
Columbus, Ohio, USA

Jorge Vidaurre, M.D.
Division of Neurology
Nationwide Children's Hospital and The Ohio State University
Columbus, Ohio, USA

Rebecca Wallihan, M.D.
Division of Infectious Diseases
Nationwide Children's Hospital and The Ohio State University
Columbus, Ohio, USA

Pedro Weisleder, M.D., Ph.D.
Division of Neurology
Nationwide Children's Hospital and The Ohio State University
Columbus, Ohio, USA

Janine Penfield Winters, M.D.
Division of Palliative Care
Nationwide Children's Hospital and The Ohio State University
Columbus, Ohio, USA

1

DIAGNOSIS AND CLASSIFICATION OF SEIZURES AND EPILEPSY SYNDROMES

Jorge Vidaurre and Anup Patel

Introduction

An epileptic seizure is the clinical manifestation (symptoms and signs) of excessive and hypersynchronous, usually self-limited, activity of neurons in the cerebral cortex. The term seizure does not imply a specific diagnosis. Instead, it defines a clinical event. Epilepsy, on the other hand, is defined as a chronic disorder characterized by recurrent (more than two) unprovoked seizures. Epilepsy is a diagnosis. Furthermore, when associated with specific EEG abnormalities and patient characteristics, epilepsy can be considered a syndrome.

The first step in the evaluation of a patient with a possible seizure is to confirm the event was indeed an epileptic seizure, as multiple disorders may manifest through events that mimic a seizure (Table 1). The clinical history remains the cornerstone of the diagnostic work-up. It is important to gather information about the events that occurred before, during, and after the episode. The neurological examination may be normal, but focal abnormalities suggest a structural brain lesion as the etiology of the seizures. According to the practice guidelines set forth by the American Academy of Neurology and the Child Neurology Society, laboratory tests have limited usefulness in the evaluation of a patient who had a first seizure.

Division of Child Neurology, Nationwide Children's Hospital and The Ohio State University, Columbus, Ohio, USA

Table 1. Non-epileptic paroxysmal events in children.

- Breath-holding spells
- Syncope
- Night terrors
- Sandifer syndrome or gastroesophageal reflux disease
- Benign paroxysmal vertigo of childhood
- Prolonged QT syndrome
- Rage attacks
- Spasmus nutans
- Tics, stereotypies, and movement disorder
- Psychogenic non-epileptic seizures

A lumbar puncture is reserved for cases where a central nervous system infection is suspected.

The electroencephalogram (EEG) is an important component of the diagnostic work-up, especially for patients who had an unprovoked event or for those in whom the event was of focal origin. As indicated above, interpretation of the EEG may help in the classification of an epilepsy syndrome. The EEG should, ideally, be recorded following a night of sleep deprivation. Such a measure increases the likelihood of recording EEG activity during drowsiness and sleep, which can increase the possibility of detecting abnormal discharges. An EEG where brain activity during these two states is not recorded would be considered to be an incomplete study.

Radiological studies, either a CT of the head or an MRI of the brain are indicated in most patients who present with partial seizures or if suspicion of a focal lesions exists. If available, a brain MRI is preferred as the resolution of the images is far superior to that which can be obtained through a CT scan of the head. If the event was preceded by head trauma, a head CT is the test of choice as it can be obtained expeditiously.

As indicated above, epilepsy is defined as two or more unprovoked seizures. After making the diagnosis of epilepsy, classifying the seizure and thus a specific epilepsy syndrome helps guide the treatment plan. In this chapter, the classification published by the Commission on Classification and Terminology of the International League Against Epilepsy (ILAE) 1981 and 1989 was used. This classification is under current review, so it is our intention not to focus on the classification but on specific clinical and EEG characteristics of well-defined epilepsy syndromes (electroclinical syndromes by the new proposed terminology, see Table 4). The first step in seizure classification is to differentiate between generalized and partial (focal) seizures. Generalized seizures involve simultaneous activation of bi-hemispheric cortical regions, and are almost always accompanied by impairment of consciousness. When motor manifestations are present, they are usually symmetric and affect both sides of the body (Table 2). A generalized epilepsy syndrome may have different types of generalized seizures (Table 3).

Table 2. International league against epilepsy (ILAE) classification of seizures.

ILAE classification of focal (partial, local) seizures

Clinical seizure type	**EEG seizure type**	**EEG interictal expression**
A. **Simple focal seizures (consciousness not impaired)**	Local contralateral discharge starting over the corresponding area of cortical representation	Local contralateral discharge
1. With motor signs. a. Focal motor without march b. Focal motor with march (Jacksonian) c. Versive d. Postural e. Phonatory (vocalization or arrest of speech)		
2. With somatosensory or special-sensory symptoms (simple hallucinations, e.g. tingling, light flashes, buzzing). a. Somatosensory b. Visual c. Auditory d. Olfactory e. Gustatory f. Vertiginous		
3. With autonomic symptoms or signs (including epigastric sensation, pallor, sweating, flushing, piloerection, and pupillary dilatation).		
4. With psychic symptoms (disturbance of higher cerebral function). These symptoms rarely occur without impairment of consciousness and are		

(*Continued*)

Table 2. (*Continued*)

Clinical seizure type	EEG seizure type	EEG interictal expression
much more commonly experienced as complex focal seizures. a. Dysphasic b. Dysmnesic (e.g. déjà-vu) c. Cognitive (e.g. dreamy states, distortions of time sense) d. Affective (fear, anger, etc.) e. Illusions (e.g. macropsia) f. Structured hallucinations (e.g. music, scenes)		
B. Complex focal seizures (with impairment of consciousness; may sometimes begin with simple symptomatology) 1. Simple partial onset followed by impairment of consciousness a. With simple focal features (Al to A4) followed by impaired consciousness b. With automatisms 2. With impairment of consciousness at onset a. With impairment of consciousness only b. With automatisms	Unilateral or, frequently, bilateral discharge, diffuse or focal in temporal or fronto-temporal regions	Unilateral or bilateral generally asynchronous focus; usually in the temporal or frontal regions
C. Focal seizures evolving to secondarily generalized seizures (this may be generalized tonic-clonic, tonic or clonic) (above discharges become secondarily and rapidly generalized) 1. Simple focal seizures (A) evolving to generalized seizures 2. Complex focal (B) evolving to generalized seizures 3. Simple focal seizures evolving to complex focal seizures evolving to generalized seizures		

From: The Commission on Classification and Terminology of the International League against Epilepsy.

(*Continued*)

Table 2. (*Continued*)

ILAE classification of generalized seizures (convulsive and non-convulsive)		
Clinical seizure type	**EEG seizure type**	**EEG interictal expression**
A1. Absence seizures a. Impairment of consciousness only b. With mild clonic components c. With atonic components d. With tonic components e. With automatisms f. With autonomic components *(b through f may be used alone or in combination)*	Usually regular and symmetrical 3 Hz but may be 2–4 Hz spike-and-slow wave complexes and may have multiple spike-and-slow wave complexes. Abnormalities are bilateral	Background activity usually normal although paroxysmal activity (such as spikes or spike-and-slow wave complexes) may occur. This activity is usually regular and symmetrical
A2. Atypical absence seizures May have: a. Changes in tone which are more pronounced than in A1 b. Onset and/or cessation which is not abrupt	EEG more heterogeneous, may include irregular spike-and-wave complexes. Fast activity or other paroxysmal actions. Abnormalities are bilateral but often irregular and asymmetrical	Background usually abnormal paroxysmal activity (such as spikes or spike-and-slow wave complexes) frequently irregular and asymmetrical
B. Myoclonic seizures Myoclonic jerks (single or multiple)	Polyspike and wave or sometimes spike and wave or sharp and slow waves	Same as ictal
C. Clonic seizures	Fast activity (10 Hz or more) and slow waves or occasional spike and wave patterns	Spike and wave or polyspike and wave discharges
D. Tonic seizures	Low voltage fast activity or a fast rhythm 9–10 Hz or more decreasing in frequency and increasing in amplitude	More or less rhythmic discharges of sharp and slow waves, sometimes asymmetrical, background is often abnormal for age

(*Continued*)

Table 2. (*Continued*)

E. Tonic-clonic seizures	Rhythm at 10 Hz or more decreasing in frequency and increasing in amplitude during tonic phase. Interrupted by slow waves during clonic phase	Polyspike and waves or spike and wave or, sometimes, sharp- and slow-wave discharges
F. Atonic seizures (astatic) *Combinations of the above may occur, e.g. B and F, B and D*	Polyspikes and wave or flattening or low-voltage fast activity	Polyspikes and slow wave

From: The Commission on Classification and Terminology of the International League against Epilepsy.

Table 3. Epilepsy classification table. The International League against Epilepsy classification of epilepsies and epileptic syndromes.

I. Localization-related (focal, local, partial) epilepsies and syndromes

A. Idiopathic (with age-related onset). At present, two syndromes are established:
   1. Benign childhood epilepsy with centro temporal spikes
   2. Childhood epilepsy with occipital paroxysms

B. Symptomatic. This category comprises syndromes of great individual variability.

II. Generalized epilepsies and syndromes

A. Idiopathic (with age-related onset, in order of age appearance)
   1. Benign neonatal familial convulsions
   2. Benign neonatal convulsions
   3. Benign myoclonic epilepsy in infancy
   4. Childhood absence epilepsy (pyknolepsy, petit mal)
   5. Juvenile absence epilepsy
   6. Juvenile myoclonic epilepsy
   7. Epilepsy with grand mal seizures on awakening

B. Idiopathic, symptomatic, or both (in order of age of appearance)
   1. Infantile Spasms
   2. Lennox Gastaux
   3. Epilepsy with myoclonic-astatic seizures
   4. Epilepsy with myoclonic absences

C. Symptomatic
   1. Nonspecific cause, early myoclonic encephalopathy
   2. Specific syndromes. Epileptic seizures may complicate many disease states. Under this heading are included those diseases in which seizures are a presenting or predominant feature.

(*Continued*)

Table 3. (*Continued*)

III. Epilepsies and syndromes undetermined as to whether they are focal or generalized

A. With both generalized and focal seizures
   1. Neonatal seizures
   2. Severe myoclonic epilepsy in infancy
   3. Epilepsy with continuous spikes and waves during slow-wave sleep
   4. Acquired epileptic aphasia (Landau-Kleffner syndrome)

B. Without unequivocal generalized or focal features

IV. Special syndromes

A. Situation-related seizures
   1. Febrile convulsions
   2. Seizures related to other identifiable situations, such as stress, hormones, drugs, alcohol, or sleep deprivation

B. Isolated, apparently unprovoked epileptic events
C. Epilepsies characterized by the specific modes of seizures precipitated
D. Chronic progressive epilepsia partialis continua of childhood

From: The Commission on Classification and Terminology of the International League Against Epilepsy.

Partial seizures affect only one portion of the brain. Hence, they usually have manifestations that involve only one body segment, and are not always associated with loss of consciousness. There are three subtypes of partial seizures: simple partial, complex partial and partial seizures with secondary generalization (Table 2). Simple partial seizures affect one portion of the brain, and consciousness is not affected. In contrast, complex partial seizures are associated with alteration of consciousness. Finally, partial seizures can become generalized. In such instances, the seizure focus is found in one brain hemisphere and then spreads to involve both hemispheres.

Idiopathic Generalized Epilepsy

A 15-year-old boy is evaluated in the emergency department for the chief complaint of a possible seizure. The event reportedly occurred at 9:00 a.m., immediately after the patient woke up from sleep. The episode is described as sudden onset of body stiffening followed by generalized tonic-clonic movements of the body and upward eye deviation. The event lasted 2 minutes. Subsequently, the youngster remained drowsy for a few hours; he has no recollection of the event. On further questioning, the patient indicates having experienced bilateral arm jerks usually early in the morning. On a few instances, also in the morning, he would drop objects held in his hands. Finally, the boy's classmates have reported to the teachers that occasionally, the boy appeared confused and unresponsive during the school day. The boy denies using substances of abuse or having experienced head trauma. There is no history of developmental delay or academic difficulties. The family medical history is remarkable for seizures in a maternal cousin whose events became evident at the age of 13 years. The general neurological examination, complete blood count, and complete metabolic panel are within normal limits. The young man's EEG has evidence of 4–6-Hz generalized spike- and polyspike-wave discharges activated by photic stimulation. Based on the clinical history and EEG abnormalities, it is determined that the boy has three seizure types: generalized tonic-clonic seizures, myoclonic seizures, and absence seizures. He is diagnosed with juvenile myoclonic epilepsy (JME).

Discussion

In the abovementioned case, the patient was diagnosed with JME. JME is an epilepsy syndrome that becomes evident during puberty. Juvenile myoclonic epilepsy accounts for 5–10% of all epilepsy cases. Three seizures types can be associated with this syndrome: myoclonic jerks, generalized tonic-clonic seizures, and absence seizures. Myoclonic jerks usually affect the upper extremities, are not associated with alteration in consciousness, and mostly occur soon after waking up from sleep. The patient may drop objects they hold in their hands, which may make some confuse the jerks with clumsiness. Two questions worth asking when eliciting this history are:

(1) When you brush your teeth in the morning, does the toothbrush occasionally flinch out of your hand?
(2) When writing during the first part of the school day, does your pen ever fly out of your hand?

Generalized tonic-clonic seizures are observed in almost 90% of patients with JME. They are usually the first symptom that makes the patient seek medical attention. The events also tend to occur in the morning. Absence seizures are present in approximately one-third of patients with JME. Since these are not as frequent, they may go unrecognized. In patients with JME, sleep deprivation and alcohol intake can precipitate seizures. The EEG of patients with JME reveals generalized 4–6-Hz spike- and polyspike-wave discharges. Photosensitivity is evident on the EEG in approximately 40% of patients. Rarely, seizures can be precipitated by environmental stimuli such as watching television, playing videogames, or looking at sunlight shining through evenly spaced trees. See Figure 1.

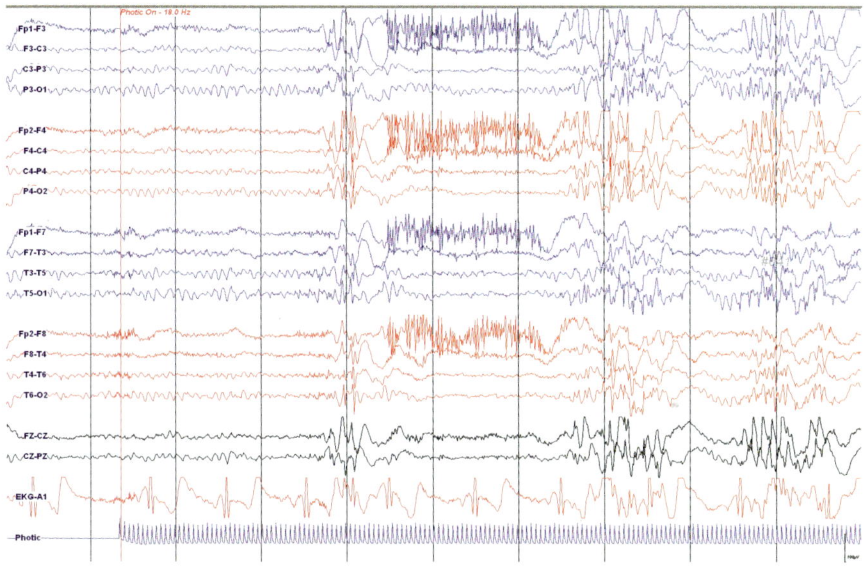

Figure 1. A 16-year-old patient with diagnosis of JME. EEG showing generalized polyspikes activated by fast photic stimulation. This was accompanied by cluster of myoclonus, followed by a GTC seizure.

Other idiopathic generalized syndromes that share similar seizure types are:

Childhood absence epilepsy

The age of onset of childhood absence epilepsy (CAE) is between 4 and 10 years of age, with a peak incidence of 6–7 years. The condition is slightly more prevalent in girls than in boys. Absence seizures are the predominant type in patients with CAE. Absence seizures consist of sudden alteration in the level of awareness lasting a few seconds; immediately thereafter, the patient regains consciousness. Absence seizures may occur hundreds of times a day, and can be precipitated by hyperventilation. Rarely, generalized tonic-clonic (GTC) seizures may be seen in patients with CAE, usually during adolescence. Remission of CAE is expected in approximately 80% of patients. The classical EEG findings in patients with CAE are those of normal background activity with ictal activity consisting of generalized, rhythmic 2.5–3.5-Hz spike-wave discharges (Figures 2a and 2b).

Juvenile absence epilepsy

Patients with juvenile absence epilepsy (JAE) are older than those with CAE. The peak incidence of JAE is 10–12 years of age. Patients who have JAE experience

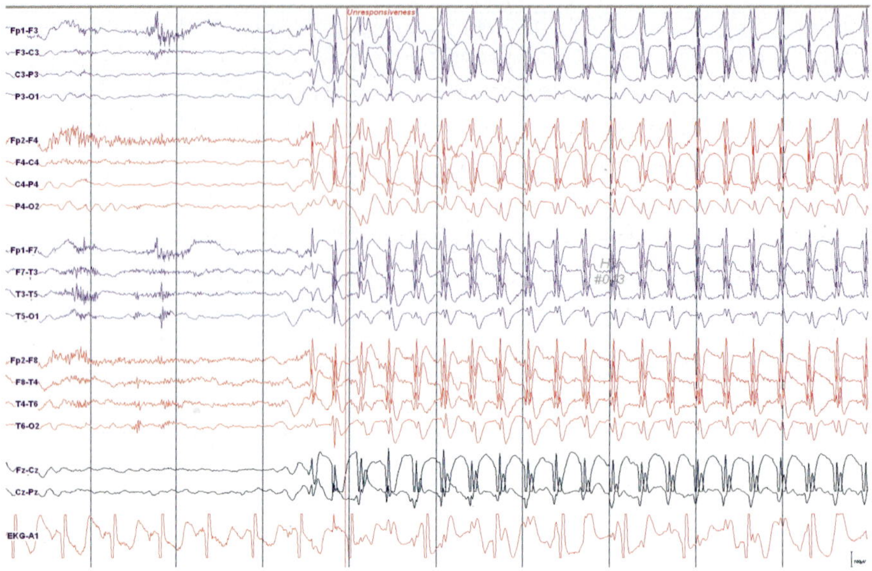

Figure 2a. An 8-year-old girl with sudden onset of generalized 3-Hz spike-wave discharges. Patient had behavioral arrest, staring and unresponsiveness.

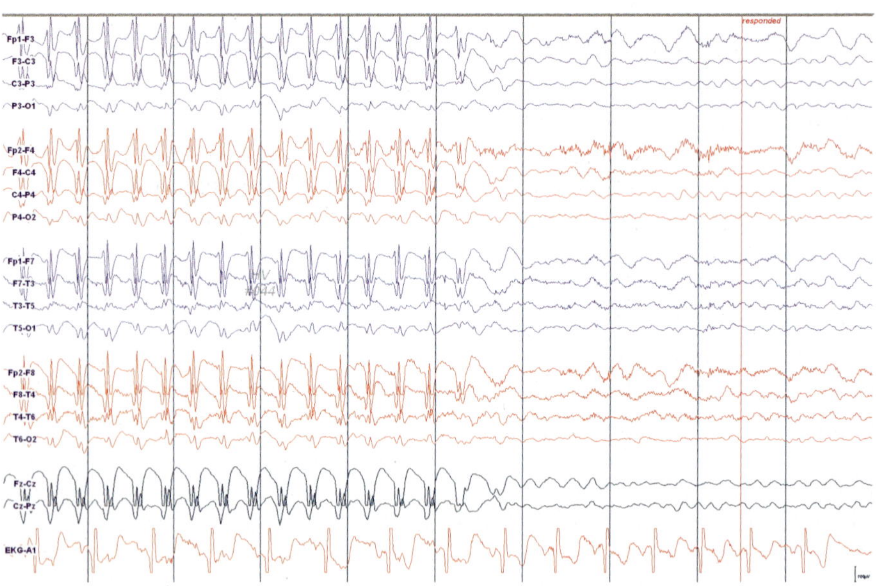

Figure 2b. Same patient as above. Sudden termination of the generalized discharges. EEG background activity returned immediately to baseline.

absences that are less frequent than in CAE and cause less impairment of consciousness. The majority of patients also have GTC seizures; these occur predominantly upon waking up from sleep. The EEG of patients with JAE consists of a normal background and interspersed generalized spike-wave discharges at faster frequencies than those observed in patients with CAE.

Epilepsy with generalized tonic-clonic seizures on awakening (Epilepsy with generalized tonic-clonic seizures alone under the new terminology)

In this epilepsy syndrome, the main seizure type is GTC. As the name implies, the events are predominantly seen in the morning soon after waking up from sleep. The seizures are infrequent and the EEG is characterized by generalized spikes- or poly-spike-wave discharges.

Symptomatic Generalized Epilepsy

The parents of a 6-month-old boy bring him to the pediatrician's office for episodes consisting of "body bends" accompanied by upward eye deviation. These episodes started a few weeks prior and were initially considered to be secondary to gastroesophageal reflux. The episodes have become more frequent, and they occur in clusters. The episodes are more common during drowsiness, sleep, and immediately after waking-up from sleep. The child cries after every episode; and the mother reports the boy being less responsive to the verbal and tactile stimulation after an event. The patient is referred to the neurology clinic for evaluation. The boy's physical examination, including Wood's lamp-assisted evaluation of the skin is unremarkable. Interpretation of the boy's EEG reveals a pattern consistent with hypsarrhythmia. The clinical events captured are consistent with flexor infantile spasms. MRI of the brain is deemed to be within normal limits. After a trial of IV pyridoxine where no changes in the EEG pattern are evident, the patient is prescribed a regiment of intramuscular injections of adrenocorticotropin hormone (ACTH). A few days later, the spasms stop and the EEG pattern normalizes.

Discussion

Infantile spasms (IS) are part of the symptomatic generalized epilepsy syndromes or epileptic encephalopathies. Infantile spasms consist of brief seizures, usually occurring in clusters during periods of drowsiness. The spasms may be "flexor" that is, flexion at the head, trunk and arms (Salaam or jackknife attacks).

The spasms may also be "extensor", that is, arms extended and contraction of the back's muscles. Some patients may have both types. At times, the muscle contractions may be followed by a cry. If left untreated or if treatment is delayed, children may develop permanent cognitive impairment.

The EEG tracing of patients with IS is characterized by disorganized high amplitude background activity associated with multifocal spikes. This pattern is known as hypsarrhythmia. During the spasms, an electrodecremental response consisting of sudden attenuation of the EEG background activity, occasionally preceded by fast rhythms, may be seen. Focal features can be observed during the clinical seizure or on the EEG. Those findings suggest the presence of a structural or focal lesion.

Onset of IS is approximately at 6 months of age. Up to a third of patients with IS have brain cortical migration defects such as those seen in patients with tuberous sclerosis complex. Therefore, it is especially important to do a thorough skin examination of patients with IS. Hypoxic ischemic encephalopathy and inborn errors of metabolism are also potential causes of IS. In 5–10% of patients with IS, the cause remains unknown (cryptogenic). Patients with cryptogenic infantile spasms have the best response to pharmacological treatment; especially if the treatment is started before signs of developmental delay become evident. Patients with IS may be diagnosed as having West syndrome. This condition consists of a triad including infantile spasms, hypsarrhythmia, and developmental delay. The triad of West syndrome was originally described in 1841 by Dr. West who observed these findings in his own son (Figures 3a and 3b).

Other syndromes to consider in this category are:

Lennox-Gastaut syndrome

Lennox-Gastaut syndrome (LGS) is another symptomatic generalized epilepsy syndrome. LGS is one of the catastrophic epilepsy syndromes. It consists of a triad of seizures of multiple types, mental retardation, and slow spike-and-wave discharges on the EEG. The different seizure types in LGS include axial tonic (the most common type observed in the syndrome), atonic, myoclonic, atypical absences, and tonic-clonic seizures. Patients with LGS may experience hundreds of events a day. Status epilepticus is commonly seen in patients with LGS; it can present as periods of obtundation that can last days, and which may be refractory to pharmacological treatment. Commonly, patients with LGS have mental retardation, autistic features, or abnormal behaviors. The EEG of patients with LGS is characterized by bursts of slow spike-and-wave discharges (frequency less than 2.5 Hz). During a tonic

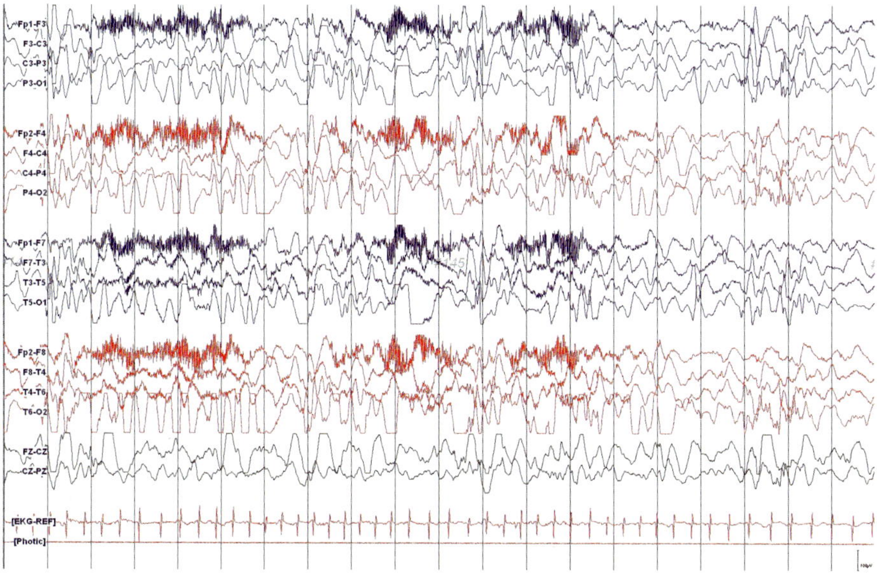

Figure 3a. A one-year-old patient with history of infantile spasms. EEG during wakefulness revealed high amplitude disorganized background with multifocal spike-wave discharges consistent with hypsarrhythmia.

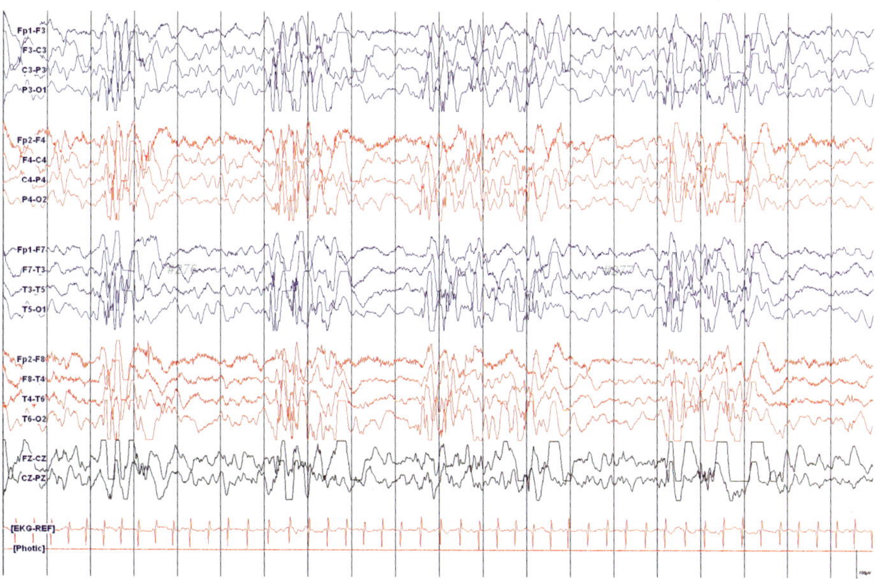

Figure 3b. Same patient as above. During sleep, the high amplitude spikes adopted a "grouping tendency", creating the impression of a discontinuous pattern.

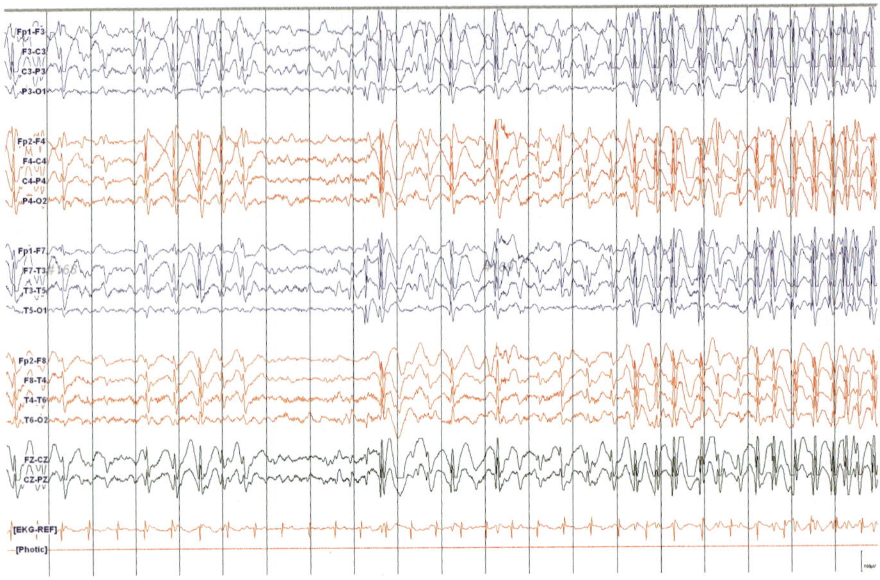

Figure 4. An 8-year-old patient with clinical picture consistent with Lennox-Gastaut syndrome. EEG showing slow background activity with intermittent frequent bursts of diffuse 1.5-Hz slow spike-wave discharges greatly activated by sleep.

axial seizure, the EEG of patients with LGS consists of fast 10–20-Hz activity which may be associated to attenuation of the overall electrical activity. Seizure control in patients with LGS is often difficult (Figure 4).

Myoclonic astatic epilepsy or epilepsy with myoclonic astatic seizures (Epilepsy with myoclonic atonic seizures under the new terminology)

Myoclonic astatic epilepsy (MAE) is another symptomatic generalized epilepsy syndrome. MAE may be difficult to differentiate from LGS. Patients with MAE present with generalized seizures, including: myoclonic, atonic, absence, tonic-clonic and tonic seizures. Episodes of status epilepticus with "minor seizures" consisting of myoclonus, drop attacks and absences can occur. In MAE, seizure severity varies from head drops to severe falls. The onset of MAE is between 18 months and 5 years of age. In contrast to children with LGS, patients with MAE usually have normal cognition. The outlook for seizure control and preservation of cognitive development is more favorable for patients with MAE than for those with LGS. The EEG of patients with MAE may have normal background activity with occasional generalized spikes and polyspike-wave discharges (Figure 5).

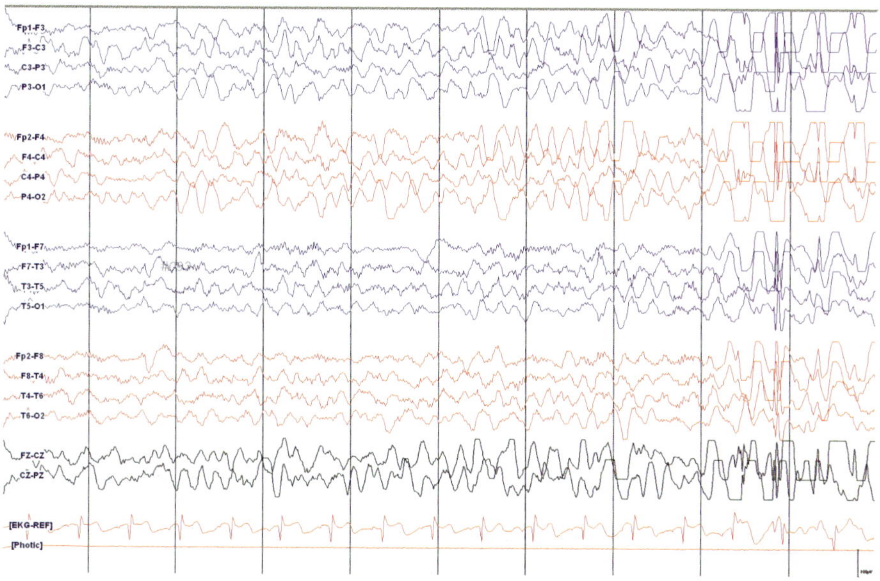

Figure 5. A 3-year-old patient with explosive onset of myoclonus, drop attacks and atypical absences. As the disorder progressed, slowing of background activity with rhythmic theta was observed. Intermittent bursts of generalized spike-wave discharges were also present.

There are other specific syndromes that deserve special consideration: Severe myoclonic epilepsy in infancy (SMEI)

From the standpoint of seizure origin SME, also known as Dravet syndrome is classified as "undetermined." The events may have both focal and generalized origin. SME was described by Charlotte Dravet in 1978. At the time of diagnosis, patients with SMEI are usually less than 1 year old. Seizure types seen in patients with SMEI include: unilateral clonic or generalized tonic-clonic seizures. Generally the first episodes are febrile convulsive seizures, but later afebrile seizures are also present. As the illness evolves, patients with SME may experience myoclonic, atypical absence, and partial seizures. The seizures in SME may be bilateral or asymmetric. At times, seizure migration from one hemisphere to the other can occur. Patients with SME may experience status epilepticus. Developmental delay, which becomes evident after seizure onset, is usually seen by 2 years of age. At the onset of the disease, the EEG of patients with SME can be normal. It may then evolve and have signs of generalized, focal or multifocal abnormal discharges. Severe myoclonic epilepsy in infancy is caused mainly by mutations in the voltage-gated sodium ion channel gene (SCN1A). The etiology, however, may be more complex as not all patients with SME have this genetic trait.

Epilepsy with Continuous Spike-and-Wave Discharges during Slow-Wave Sleep (CSWS) or Encephalopathy with Electrical Status Epilepticus during Slow-Wave Sleep (ESES)

According to the International League Against Epilepsy (ILAE) some epilepsy syndromes remain unclassified (Table 3). One such epilepsy syndrome is that of CSWS which represents an epileptic encephalopathy accompanied by multiple seizures types, including simple and complex partial, bilateral clonic, tonic-clonic, absence, and atonic seizures. The characteristic EEG of patients with CSWS consists of diffuse spike-wave discharges during 85% or more of the time the patient is in slow-wave sleep during three or more recordings over at least 1 month. Recently, however, less strict criteria have been proposed. The abnormal discharges on the EEG of patients with CSWS may have frontal predominance. In addition to seizures, patients with CSWS exhibit developmental regression with behavior disturbances, aggression or even psychotic symptoms can occur. Furthermore, motor impairment in the form of apraxia, dystonia, and ataxia has been considered part of CSWS. Structural abnormalities on brain MRI have been reported in up to 60% of patients with CSWS. These focal abnormalities are assumed to be the cause behind rapid secondary bisynchrony seen in patients with CSWS. Rapid secondary bisynchrony refers to the rapid generalization of epileptiform abnormalities (Figures 6a and 6b).

Landau Kleffner syndrome

Landau Kleffner syndrome (LKS) is an epilepsy syndrome that shares some EEG features with CSWS. The EEG of patients with LKS shows diffuse epileptiform abnormalities. During slow-wave sleep, the EEG may have evidence of electrographic status epilepticus. Spike discharges on the EEG of patients with LKS are predominately observed in the temporal regions and are usually bilateral. The clinical manifestations of LKS are consistent with an acquired epileptic aphasia in an otherwise developmentally normal child. As the disease progress, verbal auditory agnosia with difficulty understanding spoken words followed by arrest of speech becomes evident. Clinical seizures are present in 70–80% of patients with LKS; however, they occur infrequently. Approximately 50% of patients with LKS eventually develop permanent and severe impairment of speech (Figures 7a and 7b).

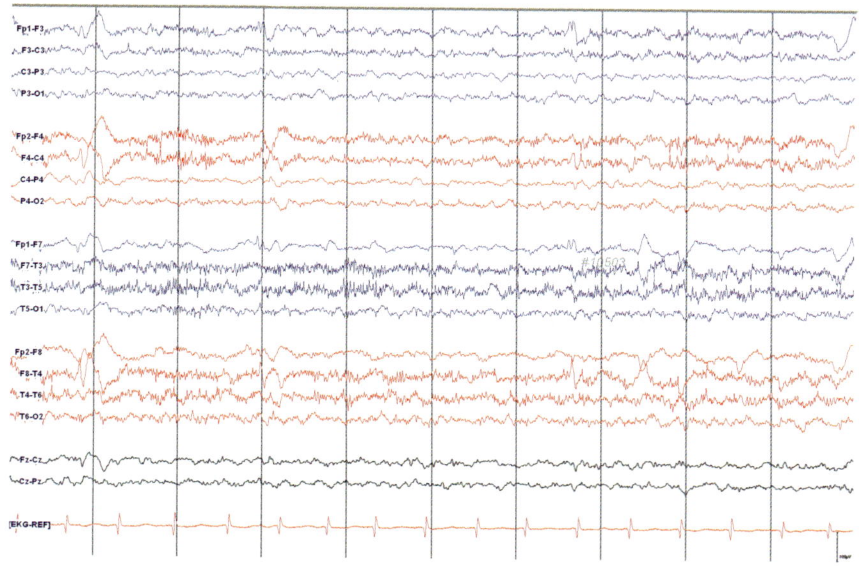

Figure 6a. An 8-year-old patient with history of atypical absence seizures, multiple episodes of "obtundation" and severe behavior problems. Background EEG during wakefulness showed only occasional epileptiform discharges.

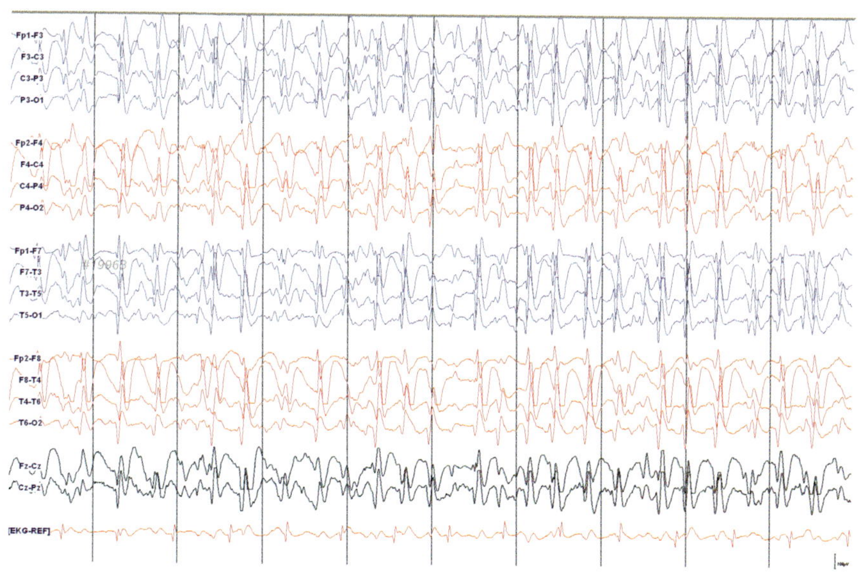

Figure 6b. Same patient as above. During sleep, the epileptiform discharges are highly activated, occupying 100% of the slow sleep record, consistent with "electrical status epilepticus during slow wave sleep".

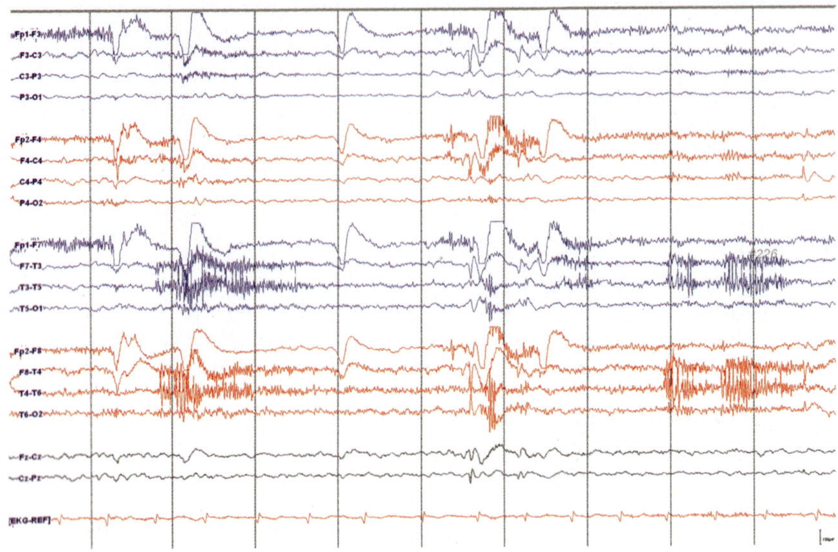

Figure 7a. A 6-year-old patient with "auditory verbal agnosia" and behavioral deterioration. EEG during wakefulness shows normal background with occasional bilateral centro-temporal spikes.

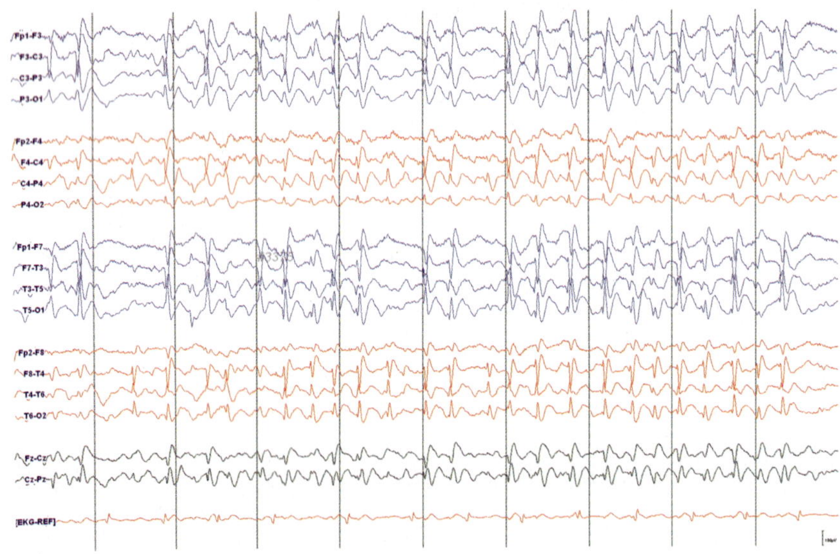

Figure 7b. Same child as above. During sleep, the spikes were greatly activated consistent with "ESES". The epileptiform discharges have left side predominance, involving mainly the central-mid temporal region.

Focal Idiopathic Epilepsy

A 6-year-old boy is evaluated in the emergency department for the chief complaint of possible seizure. At approximately 4:00 a.m., the boy's parents noticed he was standing at the threshold of their room. The left side of the boy's face was twitching, the eyes were rapidly blinking and the left side of the mouth was drawn up. During the event, the boy could not speak. The boy, however, kept the right hand over his face trying to stop the activity. The event, which the boy remembers in its entirety, lasted approximately 40 seconds. The boy is an otherwise healthy child whose development has been unremarkable. His physical and neurological examinations are normal. The boy's EEG has evidence of right central and mid-temporal spike discharges which increase in frequency during sleep. Based on the characteristics of the events and the EEG activity, the boy is diagnosed with benign rolandic epilepsy (BRE).

Discussion

BRE is also referred to as benign epilepsy with centro-temporal spikes (BECTS). According to the ILAE, BRE is classified as one of the idiopathic, localization-related epilepsies (Table 3). BRE is one of the most common epilepsy syndromes accounting for 10–20% of all patients with epilepsy. The age of onset for BRE is between 3 and 13 years of age; with a peak incidence between 5 and 8 years of age. As a general rule, children with BRE have normal development and normal neurological examination. A brain MRI is often not necessary for the diagnosis of benign epilepsy syndromes.

Seizure types seen in patients with BRE are usually simple, sensorimotor, partial seizures which manifest as unilateral paresthesias involving the lips, tongue or gums and unilateral clonic, tonic or tonic-clonic movements of the face that may extend to the arm and leg. If the tongue and laryngeal muscles become involved during the seizure, drooling and speech arrest become evident. A patient with BRE can experience a simple partial seizure and retain consciousness. But in 20–30% of patients with BRE, the seizures may subsequently become generalized. The seizures in BRE commonly occur at night; but may also be evident while the patient is awake. The EEG of patients with BRE reveals normal background activity and stereotyped, diphasic spike-and-wave discharges affecting both centro-temporal areas of the brain. The epileptic spikes in BRE often have a horizontal dipole with maximal negativity in the central and mid-temporal areas of the brain with positivity in the frontal regions. In younger patients, the spikes on the EEG may be localized to the posterior head regions. The remission rate in BRE is approximately 80% by age 16 years. During the active phase of the disorder, attention and learning difficulties may be associated with BRE (Figure 8).

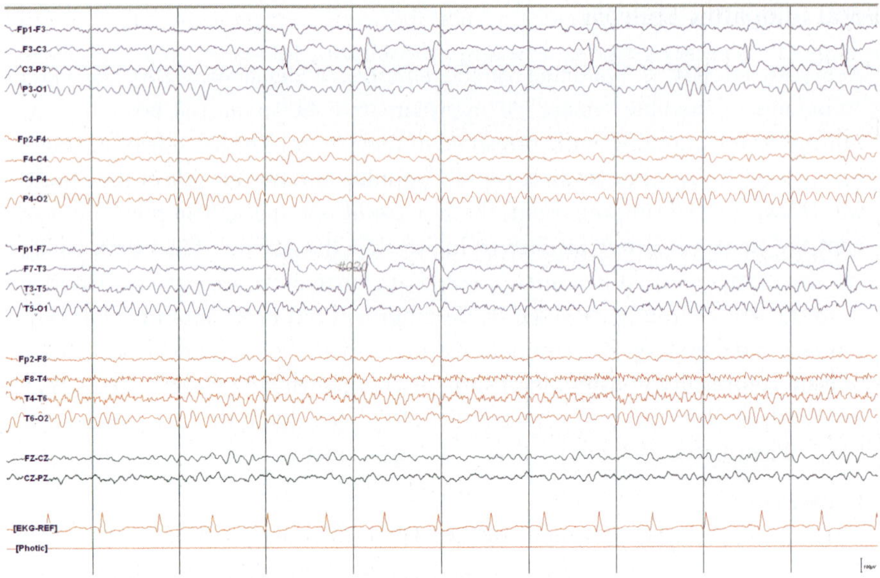

Figure 8. An 8-year-old patient with seizures consisting of "twitching" of the right side of his face and drooling, followed by clonic movements of his right arm. EEG showed left central- mid-temporal spikes (phase reversal at electrodes C3 and T3), consistent with BRE.

Panayiotopoulos type

Another idiopathic, localization-related epilepsy syndrome is benign childhood epilepsy with occipital paroxysms. The Panayiotopoulos type is a subset of benign childhood occipital epilepsy with occipital paroxysms of early onset. The Panayiotopoulos type is usually observed in children between the ages of 1 and 14 years with peak incidence at 4 to 5 years. The clinical presentation of benign childhood epilepsy with occipital paroxysms consists of autonomic symptoms (syncope-like), including nausea, emesis, pallor and pupil changes. Frequently, the seizures in the Panayiotopoulos type may last longer than 30 minutes. In the majority of patients, other symptoms such as confusion, hemi-convulsions, deviation of the eyes, or GTC seizures occur. Patients with the Panayiotopoulos type usually experience seizure remission 2 years following the onset of symptoms.

Gastaut type

The Gastaut type of idiopathic childhood occipital epilepsy affects children between 3 and 15 years of age. The seizures in the Gastaut type may include positive (visual hallucinations) or negative (blindness) visual manifestations. A migraine like headache may occur after the seizure in patients with this type epilepsy. Remission occurs in approximately 60% of patients.

References

Arzimanoglou A, *et al. Aicardi's Epilepsy in Children.* 3rd edn. Lippencott Williams & Wilkins. 2004.

Berg AT, *et al.* Revised terminology and concepts for organization of seizures and epilepsies: report of the ILAE commission on classification and terminology. *Epilepsia.* 2010.51:676–685.

Fenichel GM. *Clinical Pediatric Neurology: A Signs and Symptoms Approach.* 6th edn. Saunders Elsevier. 2009.

Glauser TA, *et al.* Ethosuximide, Valproic acid, and lamotrigine in childhood absence epilepsy. *N Engl J Med.* 2010.362:790–799.

Grunewald RA, *et al.* Juvenile myoclonic epilepsy: a review. *Arch Neurol.* 1993.50:594–598.

Panayiotopoulos CP, *et al.* Benign childhood focal epilepsies: assessment of established and newly recognized syndromes. *Brain.* 2008.131:2264–2286.

Panayiotopoulos CP. *The Epilepsies: Seizures, Syndromes and Management.* Oxfordshire (UK): Bladon Medical Publishing. 2005.

Scheltens-de Boer M. Guidelines for EEG in encephalopathy related to ESES/CSWS in children. *Epilepsia.* 2009.50:13–17.

Wong M, Trevathan E. Infantile spasms. *Pediatr Neurol.* 2001.24:89–98.

2

TREATMENT OF SEIZURES AND EPILEPSY SYNDROMES

Anup Patel and Jorge Vidaurre

Introduction

The risk of seizure recurrence following a single unprovoked event is approximately 30%. In patients who have had two unprovoked seizures, the risk of a third event climbs to approximately 60%. For these reasons treatment with anti-epilepsy medication for the former is rarely recommended, and highly encouraged after the later. As one would imagine, the clinical presentation and patient's characteristics aid in selecting the best therapy. Treatment options for a patient with epilepsy include: avoiding known seizure triggers, anti-epilepsy drugs (AED), the ketogenic diet, vagal nerve stimulator (VNS), and epilepsy surgery. AEDs are the cornerstone of the treatment of seizures and epilepsy syndromes. When selecting an AED, it is important to consider the seizure type, epilepsy syndrome (if known), co-morbid conditions, and medication side effects. There are many medications to choose from and new medications are currently in development. Even with the advent of new medications, it is important to note that successful treatment of seizures with the first AED chosen is only about 60%. If the first medication fails to control the seizures, the likelihood that a second one will achieve that goal drops to about 10%. If two medications fail to control the events, the likelihood of seizure control becomes 1–2%.

Division of Child Neurology, Nationwide Children's Hospital and The Ohio State University, Columbus, Ohio, USA

Juvenile Myoclonic Epilepsy

Juvenile myoclonic epilepsy (JME) is a primary generalized epilepsy syndrome that becomes evident during puberty. For details on the condition, please see Chapter 1. Three seizures types are associated with JME: myoclonic jerks, generalized tonic-clonic seizures and absence seizures. Major triggers for JME include sleep deprivation and alcohol use. Rarely, seizures can be precipitated by environmental stimuli such as watching television, playing video-games, or looking at sunlight shining through evenly spaced trees. Medications used to treat JME include: valproate, levetiracetam, lamotrigine, topiramate, zonisamide, and clonazepam.

Valproic acid

Although, no randomized controlled trial to determine the optimal treatment for JME has been completed, valproate has long been considered to be the treatment of choice for the condition. Valproate is also known by the names of valproic acid, Depakote, Depekene, Depacon, Depakote XR, and Stavzor. The start-up dose of valproate is 10 mg/kg/day in 2–4 divided doses. Based on seizure control, the dose is slowly titrated up to a range of 25–50 mg/kg/day. The established therapeutic range of valproate in serum is 50–100 mg/ml. Side effects of valproate are: dizziness, tremor, weight gain, nausea, and somnolence. More serious, but rare side effects include: liver toxicity, pancytopenia, and pancreatitis; monitoring for those conditions is indicated. Valproate use is contraindicated in patients with known or suspected mitochondrial disease secondary to the risk of liver failure. The risk of using valproate in young women should be weighed against the risk of potential birth defects, polycystic ovary disease, and weight gain.

Levetiracetam

Levetiracetam has also been used for the treatment of JME; its efficacy is similar to that of valproate. Levetiracetam is also known as Keppra and Keppra XR. The usual starting dose of levetiracetam is 10 mg/kg/day divided in two doses. The dose is slowly titrated to a maximum of 60 mg/kg/day. Serum levels do not correlate with efficacy or toxicity. Common side effects of levetiracetam include: irritability, somnolence, and dizziness. In rare instances, patients may experience leukopenia. Patients taking levetiracetam do not require routine laboratory testing. Levetiracetam has no known interactions with other medications.

Lamotrigine

Lamotrigine has also been used to treat JME. There are, however, case reports associating lamotrigine use and an increase in myoclonic jerks. Lamotrigine is also known as Lamictal and Lamictal XR. The usual starting dose of lamotrigine is 0.6 mg/kg/day divided in two doses. If the patient is already taking valproate, the usual starting dose is 0.15 mg/kg/day in two divided doses. To avoid the risk of Stevens-Johnson rash, a very slow titration of lamotrigine is recommended. The eventual target dose of lamotrigine is 2–10 mg/kg/day divided in two doses. As just indicated, the most serious side effect of lamotrigine is Stevens-Johnson rash. Common side effects of lamotrigine include a milder rash, nausea, and insomnia.

Topiramate

Based on a few case reports and retrospective studies, topiramate has been deemed to be effective in the management of JME. Topiramate is also known as Topamax. The usual starting dose is 1–2 mg/kg/day divided in two doses. The maximum dose of Topamax is 10 mg/kg/day. Common side effects of topiramate include somnolence, and impairment in cognition described by patients as "slow thinking" or word-finding difficulties, appetite suppression, anhidrosis, and nausea. Serious by rare side effects include the formation of kidney stones, and acute narrow-angle glaucoma. The latter has rarely been reported in children. Topiramate has no major known drug–drug interaction; routine blood monitoring is not indicated.

Zonisamide

Based on a few case reports and retrospective studies, zonisamide has been deemed effective in the treatment of JME. Zonisamide, however, may not be effective in controlling absence seizures. Zonisamide is also known as Zonegran. The medication is widely used for the treatment of primary generalized epilepsy in Japan. The usual starting dose is 1–2 mg/kg/day; it can be given once a day due to its long half-life. The dose of zonisamide is increased slowly to a maximum of 10 mg/kg/day. Side effects of zonisamide are similar to those of topiramate. Caution is advised when using zonisamide in patients with sulfa drug allergy, as there is a sulfonamide component to zonisamide.

Clonazepam

Clonazepam is a benzodiazepine effective in the treatment of myoclonic jerks. The medication is, however, not effective for the control of other seizure types seen in

JME. Clonazepam is also known as Klonopin. The starting dose of clonazepam is 0.01 mg/kg/day divided in two or three doses; it can be increased to a maximum of 0.3 mg/kg/day. The most common side effect of clonazepam is sedation.

Childhood Absence Epilepsy

As would be expected, the predominant seizure type in childhood absence epilepsy (CAE) is absence seizures. In 2009, the results of a multicenter trial on the efficacy and safety of medications used to treat CAE were published. The authors compared three AEDs: ethosuximide, valproate, and lamotrigine. Ethosuximide was found to be the most efficacious and have the least side effects. Valproate had similar efficacy to ethosuximide, but with a higher frequency of side effects. Lamotrigine was the least efficacious of the three. Based on this landmark study, ethosuximide is considered to be first line medication for CAE. Ethosuximide, however, is not effective for any seizure type other than absence seizures.

Ethosuximide

Ethosuximide is also known as Zarontin. The usual starting dose is 10–15 mg/kg/day divided in two doses. As needed, the dose can be increased to 50 mg/kg/day. Common side effects of ethosuximide include sedation, nausea, and appetite suppression. In rare instances, pancytopenia and liver toxicity have been reported. The therapeutic range of ethosuximide in serum is 40–100 mg/ml.

Benign Rolandic Epilepsy

Benign rolandic epilepsy (BRE) is also known as benign epilepsy with centro-temporal spikes (BECTS). Seizure types commonly seen in patients with BRE include simple and complex-partial. Strategies used to treat BRE can be similarly applied to patients with simple or complex-partial seizures of many origins. Medications used to treat partial seizures include: carbamazepine, oxcarbazepine, levetiracetam, topiramate, zonisamide, lamotrigine, phenytoin, and valproate.

Carbamazepine

Carbamazepine is also known as Tegretol, Tegretol XR, and Carbatrol. The starting dose of carbamazepine is 10–15 mg/kg/day divided in two or three doses, which depends on the formulation selected. The maximum dose of carbamazepine is 45–50 mg/kg/day. Side effects of carbamazepine include rash (Stevens-Johnson syndrome), drowsiness, ataxia, dizziness, hyponatremia, and nausea. The rash is more likely to occur in patients of Asian ancestry. Importantly, osteopenia can occur over time. Thus, monitoring of bone density should be considered. Liver toxicity, although rare, can also occur. The therapeutic range of carbamazepine in serum is 8–12 mg/ml. Carbamazepine induces its own metabolism; therefore, serum levels of the medication can decrease without any dose changes.

Oxcarbazepine

Oxcarbazepine has similar efficacy to carbamazepine and a lesser risk for side effects. The starting dose of Oxcarbazepine is 10 mg/kg/day in two divided doses. Based on seizure control, the dose may be increased to 20–60 mg/kg.

Phenytoin

Phenytoin is one of the most commonly used AEDs worldwide. Phenytoin is also known as Phenytek and Dilantin. The initial dose of phenytoin is 4 mg/kg/day divided in two or three doses which depends on the formulation selected. The maximum dose of phenytoin is 8 mg/kg/day. The side effects of phenytoin include: gum hyperplasia, nausea, ataxia, nystagmus, and sedation. In patients treated with Phenytoin, liver toxicity and osteopenia may occur. Thus, monitoring for these conditions is recommended. The therapeutic range of phenytoin in serum is 10–20 mg/ml. It is important to note that phenytoin binds to serum proteins. Therefore, hypoalbuminemia may result in falsely low phenytoin levels. In those instances, it is best to monitor "free" phenytoin level in serum; the therapeutic range is 1–3 mg/ml.

Infantile Spasms

Infantile spasms (IS) are part of the symptomatic generalized epilepsy syndromes or epileptic encephalopathies. IS consist of brief seizures, usually occurring in clusters, during periods of drowsiness. The EEG tracing of patients with IS is characterized by a pattern known as hypsarrhythmia. If left untreated, IS will progress to become an epileptic encephalopathy. Treatment of IS consist of the use of adrenocorticotropic hormone (ACTH), prednisone, vigabatrin, or topiramate. Successful treatment is evidenced by the cessation of spasms and normalization, or near normalization, of the EEG tracing.

Adrenocorticotropic hormone

Adrenocorticotropic hormone (ACTH) or Acthar gel has been the mainstay of treatment for IS. Depending on the cause of IS, treatment success is seen in 40–70% of patients. Management of IS with ACTH can follow one of two paradigms, high-dose and low-dose treatments. The high-dose treatment has been shown to be more effective than the low-dose treatment. Medication side effects and cost of the therapy, however, may play a role in selecting a treatment strategy for the patient. The high-dose treatment consists of 150 units/m^2 of ACTH per day for 2–8 weeks. ACTH treatment is usually followed by 2–4 weeks of progressively lower doses of prednisone. The low-dose treatment consists of 75 units/m^2 of ACTH, and follows the same schedule as the high-dose therapy. As indicated above, treatment success involves clinical resolution of the spasms and improvement of the EEG tracing. Thus, an EEG should be obtained following clinical resolution of the spasms. The most serious side effect of ACTH is immunosuppression. This can be complicated by overwhelming infections that may cause death. Another serious complication of the use of ACTH is the development of a Cushing response (widening pulse pressures, irregular breathing, and bradycardia). Less severe side effects of ACTH include: appetite increase, irritability, weight gain, hypertension, hyperglycemia, and edema. It is recommended that patients be monitored for these potential side effects. Most authors recommend that prior to initiating treatment with ACTH, the following be obtained: complete blood count, complete metabolic panel, vital signs, and a chest X-ray. As one vial of ACTH can cost as much as $26,000, insurance companies may be reluctant to pay for the medication. Prednisone is an alternative to ACTH. Prednisone has been found to be as effective as ACTH by some authors but not by others. Prednisone's side effects are similar to those of ACTH, but they are not as severe. The dose of prednisone for the treatment of IS is 1–2 mg/kg/day for 2–8 weeks.

Vigabatrin

Vigabatrin or Sabril was recently approved by the United States Food and Drug Administration for the treatment of IS. Vigabatrin has been shown to be especially effective in the treatment of IS in patients with tuberous sclerosis complex; treatment efficacy has been as high as 80%. Vigabatrin, however, may also be effective for IS from other causes. The recommended starting dose of vigabatrin is 15 mg/kg/day divided in two doses; the target dose of vigabatrin is 150 mg/kg/day and the treatment course lasts 8–12 weeks. A serious adverse effect of vigabatrin is peripheral vision impairment. This complication may not be reversible, and, in rare cases, can lead to progressive vision loss. It is recommended that, prior to treatment initiation, patients be evaluated by an ophthalmologist. Other common side effects of vigabatrin include appetite suppression, sedation, and nausea.

Ketogenic diet

The ketogenic diet has also been used to treat IS. The ketogenic diet is a high-fat, appropriate protein, and low-carbohydrate diet. Patients who follow the ketogenic diet develop a state call "ketosis" (high ketones bodies in the blood). Ketosis results in a reduction in the frequency of seizures. Dietary intake of all food items, food supplements, and medications must be monitored closely as changes in the diet may result in loss of efficacy. Side effects of the ketogenic diet include dehydration, immunosuppression, weight loss, hypercholesterolemia, and formation of kidney stones.

Topiramate

Topiramate has also been shown to be an effective treatment for IS, especially if the EEG reveals the patient to have "modified (less severe) hypsarrhythmia". The doses and side effects of topiramate were discussed above. Other medications which have been used for the treatment of IS with varying results include valproic acid, nitrazepam, pyridoxine, zonisamide, lamotrigine, levetiracetam, felbamate, ganaxolone, liposteroid, thyrotropin-releasing hormone, and intravenous immunoglobulin.

Lennox-Gastaut Syndrome

Lennox-Gastaut syndrome (LGS) is another symptomatic generalized epilepsy syndrome which also belongs to the group of catastrophic epilepsy syndromes — conditions which lead to progressive disturbance of cerebral function. LGS includes seizures of multiple types, mental retardation, and slow spike-and-wave discharges on the EEG. Patients with LGS may experience hundreds of seizures a day, and the events are difficult to control. Medications used to treat LGS include lamotrigine, topiramate, levetiracetam, valproate, ketogenic diet, rufinamide, and felbamate. Please refer to the information above regarding all but the last two medications.

Rufinamide

Rufinamide is approved by the United States Food and Drug Administration (FDA) as add-on therapy for LGS. The starting dose of rufinamide is 10 mg/kg/day divided in two doses. The medication can be increased to a maximum dose of 45 mg/kg/day. Side effects of rufinamide include sedation, nausea and emesis, gastrointestinal discomfort, and dizziness. Rufinamide is known to have interactions with valproate and phenobarbital. Thus, serum levels of those medications need to be monitored.

Felbamate

Felbamate effectively treats seizures in patients with LGS. The starting dose of felbamate is 15 mg/kg/day divided in three or four doses. The maximum dose of felbamate is 45 mg/kg/day. Serious and potentially life-threatening adverse effects include liver failure and bone marrow suppression. Routine monitoring for such concerning effects is recommended. Due to these serious side effects, felbamate is not routinely used for the treatment of other epilepsy syndromes. Common side effects of felbamate include appetite suppression, dizziness, and nausea.

Severe Myoclonic Epilepsy

Severe myoclonic epilepsy (SME), also known as Dravet Syndrome, is an epilepsy syndrome where seizures may have both focal and generalized origin. Seizure types seen in patients with SME include generalized, unilateral clonic, tonic-clonic seizures, myoclonic, atypical absence, and partial seizures. SME is caused by mutations in the voltage-gated sodium channel gene (SCN1A). The etiology, however, is likely to be more complex as not all patients with SME have these genetic mutations. Medications used to treat SME include valproate, topiramate, levetiracetam, clobazam and stiropental. In patients with SME, seizure control is often difficult. It is important to note that certain medications have been reported to worsen seizures in patients who have SME. These include phenytoin, carbamazepine, oxcarbamazepine, and lamotrigine.

Clobazam

Clobazam or Frisium is a medication with similar composition to clonazepam. Both medications have similar side effects profile, but clobazam is less sedating. Clobazam has been recently approved by the United States Food and Drug Administration for the treatment of patients with LG. The starting dose of clobazam is 0.5–1 mg/kg/day given either once a day or divided in two doses. The maximum dose of clobazam is 3 mg/kg/day.

Stiropental

Stiropental is also known as Diacomit. Stiropental is not available in the United States. The medication is, however, available in Europe. Stiropental is indicated in conjunction with valproate and clobazam as adjunctive therapy for refractory, generalized tonic-clonic seizures in patients with SME. The starting dose of stiropental is 10 mg/kg/day divided in two or three doses. The maximum dose of stiropental is 100 mg/kg/day. Common side effects include drowsiness, tremor, ataxia, nausea, and anorexia. Transient aplastic anemia and leucopenia have been reported.

References

Arzimanoglou A. Guerrini R, Aicardi J. *Aicardi's Epilepsy in Children*. 3rd ed. Lippencott Williams & Wilkins. 2004.

Bourgeois BFD. Chronic management of seizures in the syndromes of idiopathic generalized epilepsy. *Epilepsia.* 2003.44(Suppl. 2):27–32.

Buchanan N. The use of lamotrigine in juvenile myoclonic epilepsy. *Seizure.* 1996.5:149–151.

Fenichel GM. *Clinical Pediatric Neurology: A Signs and Symptoms Approach.* 6th ed. Saunders Elsevier. 2009.

Glauser TA, *et al.* A pilot study of topiramate in the treatment of infantile spasms. *Epilepsia.* 1998.39:1324–1328.

Glauser, *et al.* Ethosuximide, valproic acid, and lamotrigine in childhood absence epilepsy. *N Engl J Med.* 2010.362:790–799.

Sharpe DV, *et al.* Use of levetiracetam in juvenile myoclonic epilepsy. *Seizure.* 2008.17:64–68.

Shinnar E, *et al.* American Academy of Neurology and the Child Neurology Society Practice Parameter: medical treatment of infantile. *Neurology.* 2004.62:1668–1681.

Tsao CY. Current trends in the treatment of infantile spasms. *Neuropsychiatr Dis Treat.* 2009.5:289–299.

Wong M, Trevathan E. Infantile spasms. *Pediatr Neurol.* 2001.24:89–98.

3

GENERALIZED CONVULSIVE STATUS EPILEPTICUS

Jorge Vidaurre and Anup Patel

Definition

Status epilepticus (SE) is defined as a seizure lasting longer than 30 minutes. It can also be defined as a series of short-lasting seizures where, over a 30-minute period, the patient does not experience full recovery of consciousness. Practical and functional definitions of SE are currently under review. These definitions will likely include a shorter time period of seizure activity. SE is the most common pediatric neurological emergency. The annual incidence of SE in the United States is 10–58/100,000. The mortality rate for SE in the pediatric population varies from 3% to 9%, so early identification and treatment is very important. There are multiple forms of status epilepticus. In this chapter, we only address generalized convulsive status epilepticus.

Etiology

The most common trigger for SE in children is fever. The second and third most common triggers for SE in children are changes to anti-epilepsy medication's schedule, and non-adherance to the prescribed treatment. Other triggers for SE include metabolic derangement, inherited diseases, trauma, cerebrovascular accidents, and central nervous system infections (CNS), to name a few. It is also important to recognize that the most significant predictor of morbidity and mortality in SE is its etiology.

Division of Child Neurology, Nationwide Children's Hospital and The Ohio State University, Columbus, Ohio, USA.

Pathophysiology

Prolonged seizures cause excitotoxic neuronal injury. Excitotoxic injury depends on the duration of the seizure. Excitotoxic changes are transient in the beginning. As the seizure continues, however, these changes can lead to neuronal death. In addition, prolonged seizures can cause systemic changes that may further contribute to CNS injury.

SE can be divided into an early hyperdynamic phase, and a late hypodynamic phase. The hyperdynamic phase is characterized by tachycardia, hypertension, and hyperperfusion secondary to significant catecholamine release. If a seizure persists for a long time, the blood pressure and blood flow decrease (hypodynamic phase), but the metabolic requirements of the brain remain high. This combination of factors can lead to neuronal damage.

Patients with SE experience hypoventilation with subsequent hypoxemia and hypercarbia. The hypoxemia and hypercarbia are a consequence of chest-wall rigidity, and inability to cough-up pooled secretions. The hypercarbia may be complicated with the presence of neurogenic pulmonary edema. Patients with SE may also experience significant hyperpyrexia and rhabdomyolysis.

Convulsive status epilepticus is a condition that requires prompt medical intervention as it is unlikely that the seizure will come to a halt without the use of anti-epilepsy medication. The longer SE lasts, the harder it is to bring under control. This, in turn, increases the risk for morbidity and mortality. A common mistake in the management of status epilepticus is to administer sub-therapeutic doses or inappropriate anti-epilepsy drugs. In order to implement appropriate treatment, it is important that every hospital create an institutional protocol for the management of patients in SE. Institutions where protocols for SE are in place have reported a lower risk for morbidity and mortality. It is necessary that protocols for SE be developed in conjunction with specialist from the emergency department and pediatric intensive care units.

Treatment

For treatment purposes, we divide status epilepticus into three phases:

(1) Early status epilepticus
(2) Established status epilepticus
(3) Refractory status epilepticus

In the early phase of SE, assess and establish airway, breathing and circulation. Benzodiazepines continue to be the first-line treatment. Benzodiazepines can be easily administered at home or by emergency medical personal. During a clinic visit, parents of patients at risk for prolonged seizures should be given a prescription for, and trained on the use of rectal diazepam. Other home rescue treatment options are intranasal or buccal midazolam.

The benzodiazepines most readily available in the United States are:

Diazepam

A benzodiazepine that has high lipid affinity. Therefore diazepam has a rapid onset of action, but has rapid loss of anticonvulsant effect. A rectal preparation of diazepam can be used at home.

Lorazepam

Lorazepam has less lipid affinity than diazepam. Onset of action is approximately 2 minutes. The anticonvulsant effect of lorazepam lasts 6–12 hours. It can be given as an intravenous infusion or via an intramuscular injection.

Midazolam

Midazolam can be given IV. Midazolam can also be made into an aqueous solution that can be given IM. Emergency personal and parents can also be trained to give the aqueous solution intranasally or into the buccal aspect of the mouth.

If the benzodiazepines fail to control the seizure, the patient is considered to be in "established phase of SE (ESE)." Phenytoin and phenobarbital have been demonstrated to have similar efficacy for the management of ESE. Fosphenytoin (pH 8.6) is better tolerated than phenytoin (pH 12) as the latter can cause extravasation injury. Fosphenytoin, however, is more expensive and may not be available in some countries.

When a second medication fails to control SE, the patient is considered to be in the "refractory phase" of SE (RSE). Because the possibility of achieving control with a third anti-epilepsy medication is small, adult patients in RSE are treated with a pharmacological induced coma. In contrast, there is no consensus about the next step to take for the treatment of RSE in the pediatric population. Additional research is needed in order to create a standard and effective protocol for the management of RSE in children. This issue aside, some have suggested using phenobarbital before pharmacological induced coma is established. If the patient has to undergo a pharmacological induced coma, IV medications that can be used include pentobarbital, midazolam, propofol, and anesthetics.

Pentobarbital has been shown to be more effective that midazolam in achieving seizure control and preventing seizure recurrences. Pentobarbital, however, is more likely to produce hypotension than midazolam. Patients in medication-induced coma should be monitored with continuous electroencephalogram (EEG). From an electrophysiological standpoint, the goal of medication induced coma is attainment of a burst-suppression pattern.

Protocol for SE Management

The following is an example of our institution's protocol:

Nationwide Children's Hospital Protocol for Convulsive Status Epilepticus (SE) in Pediatric Patients after the Neonatal Period

Out-of-hospital management where neither intravenous not intraosseus access has been established (Early phase of SE)

1. Administer intranasal midazolam 0.2 mg/kg/dose (maximum 10 mg) or, buccal midazolam 0.2 mg/kg/dose (maximum 10 mg) or rectal diazepam 0.3 mg/kg/ dose (maximum 20 mg).

Management in the hospital or the emergency department

2. Assess respiratory status. Suction secretions. Provide supplemental oxygen. Avoid hypoxia.
3. Consider bag-valve mask ventilation.
4. Obtain IV access and check hemodynamic status. Avoid hypotension.
5. Using an expeditious method, assess the patient's blood glucose level. Draw blood for: basic metabolic panel, magnesium, phosphorus, calcium, complete blood count, and liver function tests. If the patient is known to take anti-epilepsy medications such as phenytoin, phenobarbital, carbamazepine, and valproic acid, blood levels should be measured. If indicated, toxicology screen should be ordered. If there is a possibility of a CNS infection, perform lumbar puncture once the patient is stable, but do not delay antibiotic and antiviral treatment. Obtain head CT scan for focal seizures, focal deficits, and history suggestive of trauma, bleeding disorder or infections.
6. Administer lorazepam 0.1 mg/kg IV (maximum 4 mg) over 1 minute. Monitor respiratory and hemodynamic status constantly.
7. If SE continues after 5 minutes (established phase of SE), administer fosphenytoin 20 mg PE/kg (at a rate not to exceed 150 mg PE/min).
8. If status continues 10 minutes after finishing the initial dose of fosphenytoin, administer an additional dose of 10 mg PE/kg.

9. If the patient is allergic to phenytoin, administer phenobarbital 20 mg/kg as a loading dose. Other medications that could be considered in a patient allergic to phenytoin include: valproic acid 30 mg/kg (at a rate not to exceed 150 mg/min) and levetiracetam 50 mg/kg (at a rate not to exceed 100 mg/min).
10. If status continues 10 minutes after finishing the second dose of fosphenytoin or a dose of a second-line anti-epilepsy drug, in the case of allergy to phenytoin (refractory SE), perform elective endotracheal intubation and administer phenobarbital 20 mg/kg dose, at a rate not to exceed 100 mg/min. If a decision is made in the ED not to intubate, the patient should be closely monitored for respiratory or hemodynamic deterioration. Arrange for long-term EEG monitoring if clinical seizures have stopped but mental status cannot be assessed, if there is suspicion for subclinical seizures, or if a paralytic medication is used to intubate the patient.

Management in the pediatric intensive care unit (PICU)

11. Continue hemodynamic monitoring and admit the patient to the PICU. Consider placing a central venous catheter.
12. If SE persists 5–10 minutes after the infusion of phenobarbital, initiate medication-induced coma with midazolam 0.2 mg/kg bolus (maximum 10 mg) over 2 minutes.
13. If status persists 5 minutes after the initial bolus, give an extra dose of 0.2 mg/kg and initiate a maintenance infusion at a rate of 0.1 mg/kg/hr.
14. If status persists 5 minutes after the above mentioned dose of midazolam, give extra boluses as needed or tolerated every 5–15 minutes and increase the infusion by 0.2 mg/kg/hr increments after each bolus (usual maximal dose: 2–4 mg/kg/ hour). Use IV fluids or vasopressors, if needed, to maintain adequate blood pressure.
15. Continue pharmacological coma for 24 hours after the last seizure to achieve a burst suppression pattern in the EEG.
16. Continue EEG monitoring with frequent reviews.
17. If SE persists after using maximal doses of midazolam or if the infusion is not tolerated, administer pentobarbital as a bolus dose of 5–10 mg/kg to be infused over 1 hour and start a maintenance infusion rate of 0.5–5 mg/kg/hr (the infusion can be increased by 0.25–0.5 mg/kg/hr) in order to achieve a burst suppression pattern on EEG. Stop midazolam drip if pentobarbital is used.
18. Other agents to consider include isoflurane, propofol, or ketamine. As indicated above, valproic acid and levetiracetam may also be used. Topiramate

can be given by a nasogastric tube at an initial dose of 10 mg/kg with maintenance of 5 mg/kg/day divided in two doses.

19. Continue fosphenytoin and/or phenobarbital maintenance. On a daily basis, check phenytoin and phenobarbital blood levels. The initial goal is to keep free phenytoin level between 1 and 3 mcg/ml and phenobarbital levels between 20 and 40 mg/ml.
20. If the patient remains seizure free for 24 hours, initiate weaning phase. Decrease the rate of midazolam infusion by 0.05 mg/kg/hour every 3–4 hours. If pentobarbital was used, reduce by 0.5 mg/kg/hr every 12 hours or slower, for patients who have been on pentobarbital for a long period.
21. If the patient has no further seizures, continue decreasing the medications used to induce coma until discontinued. Continue EEG monitoring for at least 24 hours after the infusion has been terminated, in order to monitor for recurrence of electrographic seizures.
22. If status recurs, reinstitute midazolam or pentobarbital coma. Wait 48 hours before the next attempt at discontinuing medications.

Protocol currently under review.

4

MANAGEMENT OF SEIZURES IN THE EMERGENCY DEPARTMENT

Kimberly Scansen

Status Epilepticus

A 9-year-old female with a history of epilepsy is brought to the emergency department (ED) by ambulance. The child is in the midst of a seizure that began 30 minutes prior. During the trip to the ED, the paramedics gave her oxygen and unsuccessfully attempted to place an intravenous (IV) catheter. The child received a dose of rectal diazepam. On the way to the hospital, the patient's generalized muscle contractions stopped briefly, but a few minutes later started once again. As the stretcher with the patient rolls through the doors of the ED, the patient is noted to have generalized tonic-clonic contractions involving all four extremities.

The patient described above is in status epilepticus because of the duration of the seizure without recovery of consciousness (> 30 minutes for a single seizure or multiple seizures without recovery of consciousness between the seizures). The initial management should focus on the ABCs: airway, breathing, and circulation. Patients in status epilepticus should be placed on oxygen; the cardio-respiratory status should be monitored continuously. An IV should be placed for medication administration. If IV access is not possible, an intraosseous needle can be placed or alternate medication administration routes must be

Division of Emergency Medicine, Nationwide Children's Hospital and The Ohio State University, Columbus, Ohio, USA considered (rectal, intramuscular, intranasal, buccal). Cessation of the seizure via pharmacological intervention as soon as possible is a priority. The longer seizures last, the more difficult it is to stop them; and the higher the morbidity and mortality. A blood glucose level should also be checked as part of the initial evaluation.

Impaired consciousness, as may be seen in patients with epilepsy, may hamper a patient's ability to protect the airway; this can result in aspiration of saliva or stomach contents. Furthermore, inadequate ventilation can lead to hypoxia, hypercarbia and respiratory acidosis. Initial airway management may include suctioning of secretions, jaw thrust maneuvers and use of a nasopharyngeal airway. Bag valve-mask ventilation may also be utilized during a seizure. If the aforementioned maneuvers are not adequate and spontaneous ventilation has not returned, intubation and mechanical ventilation would be the next logical step.

Pharmacological Management of a Seizure

Benzodiazepines are the first-line pharmacologic therapy for ongoing seizures. Lorazepam 0.05–0.1 mg/kg IV is the benzodiazepine of choice. If needed, the dose may be repeated. For a patient without IV access, rectal diazepam may be used in place of lorazepam. The dose of rectal diazepam is based on the patient's age and weight: 0.5 mg/kg for patients who are 2–5 years of age; 0.3 mg/kg for patients who are 6–11 years old; and 0.2 mg/kg for patients who are 12 years or older (maximum dose: 20 mg). Another option for patients without IV access is midazolam 0.2–0.5 mg/kg (maximum dose: 10 mg) given via intranasal or buccal routes. The authors of several studies have suggested that midazolam (intranasal or buccal) is more effective, and has fewer side effects than rectal diazepam.

If the seizure does not stop with benzodiazepines, fosphenytoin is the next medication recommended. The dose of fosphenytoin is 20 mg phenytoin equivalents (PE)/kg. Fosphenytoin can be given either intravenously or intramuscularly; however, absorption is poor with intramuscular administration. Fosphenytoin is a precursor of phenytoin that has marked advantages. Specifically, fosphenytoin causes less soft tissue damage if there is extravasation, may be given more quickly, and has a lower rate of cardiovascular side effects (hypotension, cardiac arrhythmia) than phenytoin. If the seizure persists despite a dose of fosphenytoin, the next recommended drug for the patient is phenobarbital 15–20 mg/kg IV. In the uncommon event that the previous medications do not successfully control the seizure, the patient will need to be placed in a pharmacologic coma. In this instance, the patient requires continuous EEG monitoring as well as admission to the intensive care unit.

Medications used for the acute management of seizures can cause significant respiratory depression. As additional medications are administered to terminate a seizure, the child may need endotracheal intubation and mechanical ventilation. If necessary, a paralytic agent with a short half-life should be used for intubation. After intubation, additional doses of paralytic medications should be avoided because these agents mask seizure activity and thus take away the clinical exam as a way to guide further interventions. In addition to medications commonly used for intubation, propofol can be considered. After intubation, the patient should be transitioned to other sedative medications.

Clinical History

The following is a list of questions that should be asked in the ED:

- How long did the seizure last?
- What did the seizure look like (focal, generalized, tonic, clonic etc.)?
- Does the patient have a history of epilepsy or previous seizures?
- Was the event a "typical" seizure for the patient?
- How often does the patient have seizures?
- Does the patient take anti-seizure medications?
- Has the patient been taking the anti-seizure medications as directed?
- Have there been any recent changes to the patient's medication schedule?
- Does the patient have other significant past medical history?
- Has the patient undergone neurosurgical procedures?
- Is it possible the patient might have ingested a toxic substance?
- Is there a recent history of head injury or trauma?
- What other symptoms did the patient have prior to the seizure (fever, headache, emesis, rashes, mental status changes)?
- Are there other family members with a history of a seizure disorder?

Differential Diagnosis

The differential diagnosis for a patient being evaluated in the ED for seizures should include the following categories:

(1) Infections: meningitis, encephalitis (herpes simplex or other viruses), brain abscesses, parasitic infections.
(2) Metabolic derangements: hypoglycemia, hypocalcemia, hyponatremia, inborn errors of metabolism, pyridoxine deficiency, uremia.
(3) Vascular: cerebrovascular accident, hypertensive encephalopathy, intracranial hemorrhage.

(4) Toxicological: ingestion, inhalation, exposure or withdrawal of substances of abuse.
(5) Trauma: non-accidental trauma, closed head injury.
(6) Oncological: brain tumor, metastatic disease.
(7) Neurological: epilepsy, febrile seizure.
(8) Obstetrical: eclampsia.

It is also important to consider pharmacological causes of a seizure such as a child outgrowing a weight-based dose of medication or the possibility of non-adherence to a prescribed medication schedule.

Laboratory and Radiological Tests

The patient's clinical picture dictates which tests are to be ordered. A bedside glucose should be obtained early as part of the evaluation. Obtaining serum electrolytes' levels should be considered for a patient in status epilepticus, as unresolved electrolyte abnormalities can cause refractory seizures. In the case of a prolonged seizure, the patient can develop rhabdomyolysis, hyperkalemia, hyperthermia, and hypoglycemia, each of which needs to be identified and appropriately treated.

If trauma is a concern as the etiology of the seizure, cervical-spine immobilization should be an initial priority and be maintained throughout the evaluation. An emergent CT scan of the head should be included in the evaluation of trauma as a cause of seizures. The test may also provide valuable information if oncologic, vascular and some infectious process are the etiology of the seizure.

A 2-year-old male with no significant past medical history is brought to the ED by ambulance after he suddenly became unresponsive and started "shaking all over." The child's mother reports the episode lasted 5–10 minutes; it was over by the time the paramedics arrived at the home. Upon arrival to the ED, the child is sitting up, crying and reaching for his mother. Upon further questioning, the mother relates that her son has been eating well and was acting normally prior to this episode. He has had no fever. He did not sustain any head trauma. The child's immunizations are up to date and he has been achieving developmental milestones as expected. The child has never had a seizure before and has no other medical problems. There is no family history of seizures. The child's physical examination is normal.

First Steps

As is the case with most seizures, the event stopped without intervention. There is no acute intervention necessary with regard to airway, breathing or circulation.

A post-ictal period of sleepiness (decreased responsiveness) is common after a seizure. Regardless, the situation requires that a thorough history and physical exam be completed; and the patient should be observed until he has returned to functional baseline.

Laboratory and Radiological Tests

In a child older than 6 months of age with a first time afebrile seizure who has returned to functional baseline and has no significant past medical history nor abnormal physical examination findings, there is no indication for laboratory testing. Standard laboratory tests in a case such as the one described yield little useful information. Standard of care for a patient with a first time afebrile seizure includes an EEG and imaging of the brain. The EEG does not need to be completed urgently or emergently; it can be done as an outpatient. From a radiological standpoint, MRI of the brain is the test of choice; it can also be completed non-emergently. The exception to this rule is a patient who exhibits focal deficits on physical examination or does not return to functional baseline within a few hours. In such instances, the patient should undergo emergency neuroimaging and be admitted to the hospital.

Treatment

The vast majority of children who have a seizure are unlikely to have a recurrence. Starting an anti-epilepsy drug (AED) does not prevent the development of epilepsy and there are significant potential side effects. Current recommendations are that the decision to initiate an AED include a risk/benefit analysis, and be individualized to the patient and family. This discussion is probably best undertaken by the family with their primary care provider or neurologist outside of the acute setting of an ED.

A 2-year-old male with no significant past medical history is brought to the ED by ambulance after he suddenly became unresponsive and started "shaking all over." The child's mother reports that the episode lasted 5–10 minutes; it was over by the time the paramedics arrived at the home. The seizure resolved without any intervention and the child has been sleepy ever since. Upon arrival to the ED, the child is sitting up, crying and reaching for his mother. Upon further questioning, the mother indicates that her son has had cough, rhinorrhea and chest congestion for 3 days. The boy started pulling on his ears this morning. He has been eating well and was acting normally prior to this episode. During the trip to the ED, the paramedics checked the child's temperature — it was 102.8 °F. The child's immunizations are up to date and he is developmentally appropriate.

The child has never had a seizure before. The physical examination reveals bilateral acute otitis media. Eventually, the child is diagnosed as having had a simple febrile seizure as a consequence of acute otitis media. A prescription for the boy to take amoxicillin is given to the mother, and the patient is discharged home.

The majority of febrile seizures stop without intervention. In the clinical scenario described above, the patient is awake, acting normally and no longer in the midst of a seizure. Hence, emergent interventions are not necessary. That said, the situation warrants a thorough history and physical examination to identify sources of fever which may require further treatment. Febrile seizures are the most common seizure type in young children; they are seen in 2–5% of the population. The clinical history reveals that the child has an elevated temperature in close proximity to the seizure. The authors of a recent study on febrile seizures reported that 21% of children had seizures either before or less than one hour after identification of the fever; most patients (57%) had a seizure 1–24 hours after the fever had been identified; and the remaining 22% of children had a seizure more than 24 hours after the fever was recognized. For an event to be classified as a "simple febrile seizure", it must be generalized and last less than 15 minutes. A febrile seizure lasting more than 15 minutes, one where the event was deemed to have been a focal seizure or a situation where the patient experiences more than one seizure in 24 hours is considered a "complex febrile seizure." Viral infections are a frequent cause of febrile seizures. Human herpes virus infections (HHV-6 and HHV-7) are commonly associated with febrile seizures. Risk factors for febrile seizures include: prior febrile seizure (especially before 18 months of age); family history of febrile seizures; neonatal nursery stay of more than 30 days; developmental delay; and daycare attendance. The peak incidence of febrile seizures is 18 months of age; and most patients outgrow febrile seizures by 5 years of age. As a general rule, simple febrile seizures are not associated with identifiable brain damage.

Many young patients with febrile seizures are seen in the ED; and in most instances, the seizure ends prior to arrival. Observation in the ED until the patient returns to baseline in addition to an evaluation for treatable sources of fever (i.e. otitis media, strep throat, urinary tract infection) is customary. A well appearing child with a simple febrile seizure who has a normal neurological examination may be safely discharged home. A patient who deviates from this description will likely need further evaluation and hospital admission.

Anticipatory guidance for the caregivers of a child who experienced a simple febrile seizure and is being discharged home is important. It is estimated that 30% of children who had a febrile seizure will experience a recurrence. If this occurs, parents should make sure the child cannot be injured (i.e. a fall); and they should never attempt to pry the child's mouth open. Caregivers should be counseled that medications are unlikely to prevent a febrile seizure. The authors of several studies have shown that even scheduled doses of anti-pyretic medications are ineffective in reducing the risk of febrile seizures. If a second seizure occurs within 24 hours of the initial event, the patient should be reevaluated as, by definition, the "simple febrile seizure" has now become a "complex febrile seizure."

Lumbar puncture (LP) for cerebrospinal fluid (CSF) evaluation should be considered in a patient who is less than 12 months of age. CSF evaluation is not recommended for a child older than 12 months of age, unless there is suspicion for meningitis. Children in this age range can be more difficult to examine, so careful evaluation is essential. Recommendations for an LP and CSF analysis would include: children with a complex febrile seizure, children with persistent lethargy, those who have undergone antibiotic therapy recently, or children who have concerning findings on physical or neurological examination.

A 4-day-old male is brought to the ED by his mother who is concerned about him "shaking too much." On initial evaluation, the child's vital signs are normal for age and he is drinking a bottle with milk formula. The mother reports that over the last day she has seen the child's left arm "shaking." The boy has had three or four episodes lasting 30–45 seconds. The child's parents brought him to the ED because with the last episode his face "turned blue" and he seemed limp. The mother reports the child has been eating less and seems to be tired. She has had to wake him up to eat several times in the last day. The boy was born at 39 weeks of gestation via a normal spontaneous vaginal delivery following an uncomplicated pregnancy, and went home with his mother.

Generalized, rhythmic shaking and stiffening can be readily identified as concerning for seizure activity, however this constellation of signs is less common in neonates (less than 28 days old). Neonatal seizures are often much more subtle and necessitate close observation for diagnosis. In a neonate, a seizure may present with only lip smacking, chewing motions, eye rolling, repeated blinking or staring spells. Alternatively, the child may have episodes of apnea and cyanosis. An apparent life-threatening event may be the first manifestation of a seizure.

The differential diagnosis for neonatal seizures (with some specific examples) includes:

(1) Infections: meningitis, TORCH infections, brain abscess.
(2) Metabolic derangements: hypoglycemia, hypocalcemia, hyponatremia, hypomagnesemia, inborn errors of metabolism.

(3) Vascular: cerebrovascular accidents.
(4) Toxicological: withdrawal from medications or illegal substances.
(5) Trauma: accidental and non-accidental trauma, intracranial hemorrhage.
(6) Neurological: congenital abnormalities of the central nervous system, epilepsy, hypoxic ischemic brain injury.

Encephalitis caused by herpes simplex virus is of particular concern in this age range. Undiagnosed metabolic derangements that cause seizures (hypocalcemia, inborn errors of metabolism, hypomagnesemia, pyridoxine deficiency) are more common in children less than 6 months old. Hyponatremic seizures can be seen in infants who are being fed diluted milk formula or who are given water. Congenital brain abnormalities, drug withdrawal, and perinatal hypoxic brain injury as well as traumatic brain injury (accidental and non-accidental trauma) need to be considered in this population.

Physical Examination

A neonate may have an undiagnosed congenital anomaly triggering the seizures. The physical exam can help identify stigmata of specific diseases: café-au-lait spots associated with neurofibromatosis; a port-wine stain on the face as may be seen in patients with Sturge-Weber syndrome; and ash-leaf spots as may be seen in patients with tuberous sclerosis. Macrocephaly and an enlarged fontanelle suggest increased intracranial pressure. Neonates and infants who have seizures must also be evaluated for possible trauma. Unexplained swelling of the head or bruising are findings which may point to inflicted trauma as the cause of seizures.

Laboratory and Radiological Tests

The workup for a neonate with a first seizure should include a full septic workup and a head CT. The septic workup consists of a complete blood count (CBC), a blood culture, a urine analysis, a urine culture and a lumbar puncture for CSF analysis. If there is concern for increased intracranial pressure, the head CT should be obtained before the lumbar puncture. Once obtained, the CSF should be sent for routine studies (cell count, protein, glucose and bacterial culture) as well as evaluated for HSV — ideally by polymerase chain reaction (PCR). In a neonate with seizures, antibiotic and antiviral treatment is indicated until the appropriate studies are shown to be negative. Serum glucose and electrolytes (including calcium, magnesium, and phosphorus) should be obtained. If there is concern for an inborn error of metabolism, ammonia and serum amino acids as well as urine organic acids should be checked. Traumatic injury should be strongly considered in a neonate with new onset seizures. If there is any concern for trauma, the patient needs to

Table 1. Pharmocologic treatment for status epilepticus.

Medication	Dosing	Max dosing	Ages	Route
Lorazepam	0.05–0.1 mg/kg			IV
Diazepam	0.5 mg/kg		2–5 years old	Rectal
	0.3 mg/kg		6–11 years old	Rectal
	0.2 mg/kg	20 mg	12 years or older	Rectal
Midazolam	0.2–0.5 mg/kg	10 mg		Intranasal or buccal
Fosphenytoin	20 mg/kg			Intravenous or intramuscular

have a cervical spine collar placed. In this situation the patient should also have a comprehensive trauma evaluation and the appropriate authorities (child welfare services, police, etc.) need to be notified. As a rule, a neonate who has had a seizure needs admission to the hospital for further monitoring and treatment.

References

Bui TT, Delgado CA, Simon HK. Infant seizures not so infantile: first-time seizures in children under six months of age presenting to the ED. *Am J Emerg Med.* 2002.20: 518–520.

Fleisher GR, Ludwig S, Henretig FM. *Pediatric Emergency Medicine.* 5th ed. Philadelphia: Lippincott, Williams & Wilkins. 2006.629–636, 1332–1333.

Hirtz D, Ashwah S, Berg A, *et al.* Practice Parameter: evaluating a first nonfebrile seizure in children. *American Academy of Neurology.* 2000. Available at: http://www.aan.com/professionals/practice/pdfs/gl0081.pdf

Hirtz D, Berg A, Bettis D, *et al.* Practice parameter: treatment of the child with a first unprovoked seizure. *American Academy of Neurology.* 2003. Available at: http://www.aan.com/professionals/practice/pdfs/chi_unp_sei.pdf

Holsti M, Sill BL, Firth SD, et al. Prehospital intranasal midazolam for the treatment of pediatric seizures. *Pediatr Emerg Care.* 2007.23:148–153.

Maria BL. *Current Management in Child Neurology.* 4th ed. Shelton, CT. People's Medical Publishing House. 2009.99–104, 612–617.

Marr J, Okada PJ. Seizures. In: Baren JM, Rothrock SG, Brennan JA, *et al.* (eds.) *Pediatric Emergency Medicine.* Philadelphia: Elsevier, 2008.pp. 353–359.

McIntyre J, Robertson S, Norris E, *et al.* Safety and efficacy of buccal midazolam versus rectal diazepam for emergency department treatment of seizures in children: a randomized controlled trial. *Lancet.* 2005.366:205–210.

Mpimbaza A, Ndeezi G, Staedke S, et al. Comparison of buccal midazolam with rectal diazepam in the treatment of prolonged seizures in Ugandan children: a randomized clinical trial. *Pediatrics.* 2008.121:e58–e64.

Reuter D, Brownstein D. Common emergent pediatric neurologic problems. *Emerg Med Clin North Am.* 2002.20:155–162.

5

HEADACHES IN CHILDREN AND ADOLESCENTS

Ann Pakalnis

DK is a 17-year-old girl who is evaluated for headaches which began when she was 12 years old. The headaches are happening about six times a month, and she misses school at least 2 days a month. The headaches are usually bifrontal, associated to nausea, and light and sound sensitivity. The headaches do not wake the patient up, nor are they related to her menstrual cycle. DK's mother and maternal grandmother have experienced headaches similar to those of the girl. DK's headaches last about 6 hours. She takes ibuprofen 600 mg with only partial relief. She is applying to colleges and is working part-time as a lifeguard. She skips breakfast frequently (would rather sleep) and drinks several caffeinated sodas a day, but "drinks a lot of water because her swim coach tells her to at practice." Her physical and neurological examinations are normal. Blood pressure was 110/72. Funduscopic examination was normal.

Impression

1. DK's headaches fulfill ICHD-II criteria for migraine. Nausea, frontal throbbing pain, photophobia and phonophobia, and are severe enough to miss school or go to urgent care. Family history of migraine also occurs in about 80% of patients.
2. Radiological tests are not indicated because: the physical examination is within normal limits, the headaches are long-standing, the symptoms do

Division of Child Neurology, Nationwide Children's Hospital and The Ohio State University, Columbus, Ohio, USA

not wake the patient up nor does she wake up with headaches, and there is positive family history of similar headaches.

3. Education regarding keeping a headache diary, adequate sleep, and regular meal time is important. Hydration, especially with her active exercise schedule, and refraining from caffeinated beverages is recommended.
4. Should be a good candidate for non-pharmacologic therapies if interested. Stress can worsen headaches and, with college years and young adulthood approaching, this would be an optimal time to commence such a treatment plan.
5. Her current headache abortive therapy does not seem to be adequate, and she would be an excellent candidate for a triptan. With rapid onset of action, oral rizatriptan or nasal sumatriptan or zolmitriptan, would be good options.
6. Consideration of a preventive medication should be discussed with DK and her family. Amitriptyline or topiramate may be options, depending on patient/family preference. Divalproex would generally not be recommended in an adolescent girl because of its teratogenic side effects.

Introduction

Headaches are one of the most common neurological complaints in the pediatric population. They may be indicative of a primary headache disorder, such as migraine or tension type headaches, or secondary headaches as a symptom of an organic, systemic, or neurological illness. In this chapter, I will discuss the most common primary headache disorders, such as episodic migraine, tension, and chronic daily headaches. Common secondary causes of headaches in children and adolescents will also be reviewed.

Evaluation of the Pediatric Patient with Headaches

A thorough history is paramount and should be obtained from the adolescent or with parental input in the younger patient. Factors to be delineated include onset, location and description of pain and, of course, history of other variables, such as family history of headaches, or history of head trauma with secondary headaches. Some medications may play a role in inducing headaches; examples include the neurostimulants used in attention-deficit disorder or some of the anti-epilepsy medications such as carbamazepine. Also, some disease processes may be associated with secondary headache, such as post-ictal headaches in epilepsy patients and poorly controlled hypertension.

Thorough physical and neurological examinations are crucial to exclude other disease processes. An abnormal neurological examination can identify the need for brain imaging with magnetic resonance imaging (MRI) generally being the study of choice. Funduscopic examination may help identify signs of increased intracranial pressure such as papilledema.

Lumbar puncture may be necessary if an acute infectious process is suspected. Localized headaches with viral syndromes may be suggestive of acute sinusitis, especially in patients whose headaches are positionally and unresponsive to narcotic analgesics.

Acute Headaches

The authors of recent studies have investigated the clinical presentation of children and adolescents who visit emergency departments with acute headache. Lewis *et al.* studied 150 children and teenagers from 2–18 years of age who presented to their emergency department with abrupt onset of severe headaches. The most common etiology was upper respiratory tract infection with fever (39%) followed by sinusitis (9%). Migraine was also common (18%). Serious neurological conditions were found in 15% of patients (including viral meningitis, brain tumor and intracranial hemorrhage). Two features of the headaches which have statistically significant association with serious neurological disease are: occipital location of the headaches and inability to describe the quality of the pain.

Primary Headache Disorders

Migraine headaches occur frequently in the pediatric population. Prevalence varies between 4% in younger school-aged children to nearly 20% in adolescents. Before the age of 7 years, the prevalence of migraine is higher in boys. The difference disappears some time between 8 and 11 years of age. And starting in adolescence, the prevalence of migraine is higher in young ladies.

The International Classification of Headache Disorders (ICHD-II) includes diagnostic criteria for headache disorders, both primary and secondary. These criteria are presented in Table 1. Migraine with aura occurs in 15–30% of migraineurs. Pediatric migraine differs from adult headache regarding several features. They may be shorter in duration in children, and are more frequently associated with emesis. Uncommon migraine syndromes, such as basilar migraine, with posterior fossa symptomatology including ataxia and diplopia, and hemiplegic migraine with motor weakness are infrequent. Secondary headaches need to

Table 1. International criteria for headache diagnosis, 2nd Edition, 2004.

Pediatric migraine without aura:
- (A) More than 5 attacks fulfilling features B through D.
- (B) Headache attack lasting 1 to 72 hours.
- (C) Headache has at least 2 of the following 4 features:
  - Either bilateral or unilateral (frontal/temporal) location
  - Pulsating quality
  - Moderate to severe intensity
  - Aggravated by routine physical activities
- (D) At least 1 of the following accompanies headache:
  - Nausea and/or emesis
  - Photophobia and phonophobia (may be inferred from their behavior)

Migraine with aura:
- (A) At least 2 attacks fulfilling criteria (B) below
- (B) Aura consisting of at least 1 of the following, but no motor weakness:
  - Fully reversible visual symptoms including positive features
  - Fully reversible sensory symptoms including positive features (i.e. pins and needles) and/or negative features (i.e. numbness)
  - Fully reversible dysphasic speech
- (C) At least 2 of the following:
  - Homonymous visual symptoms and/or unilateral sensory symptoms
  - At least 1 aura symptom develops gradually over 5 minutes and/or different symptoms occur in succession over 5 minutes
  - Headache begins during the aura or follows within 60 minutes

be excluded before making these uncommon diagnoses. Other causes could be vascular, posterior fossa lesions, or Todd's paralysis after a seizure event.

Therapies

After migraine is diagnosed, exacerbating factors, particularly lifestyle issues including sleep, adequate fluid intake, regular meals and exercise, and limited caffeine intake, should be discussed. Maintaining a headache diary is an important part of the treatment regimen. Co-morbid conditions, such as depression, anxiety, and sleep disorders, are common in patients with migraine, and negatively impact successful treatment outcomes. Some non-pharmacologic therapies, such as biofeedback and cognitive behavioral therapy, are reasonable treatment options; they are safe and cost-effective. Children 9-years of age or older are generally good candidates and can be cooperative with these therapies. They are usually directed by a psychologist or licensed social worker with training in these non-pharmacological options.

Acute management of migraines

Treating early in the course of the migraine attacks is very important. Regarding over-the-counter abortive therapies, ibuprofen 10 mg/kg/dose has been studied with most favorable results. It has a longer duration of action than acetaminophen (15 mg/kg/dose). Other non-steroidals, such as naproxen sodium, have not been thoroughly studied in children, but reproducible safety and efficacy data in adult patients are available.

The triptans are serotonin 1B/1D agonists which are migraine-specific abortive therapy. This class of medications dates back to 1993 when sumatriptan subcutaneous injection became available in the United States. There are now seven different triptans available (Table 2); however, only oral almotriptan has been approved by the United States Food and Drug Administration (US FDA) for use by pediatric patients.

When to use a preventive medication is a complex decision. This is generally based on frequency and disability of the symptoms. Generally, if the episodes occur at least three times a month, it may be reasonable to discuss use of a preventive medication. About 30% of children and adolescents will be candidates for a prophylactic migraine medication. Currently, the US FDA has not approved any medication for migraine prophylaxis in the pediatric population. In adults, timolol, propranolol, divalproex and topiramate are approved.

There are some good reproducible studies in the adult and pediatric population regarding naturalistic therapies. These are popular with the lay public. They are generally safe, inexpensive, do not require a prescription and are readily available. Butterbur is an herbal preparation from the petadolax plant which is

Table 2. Commonly used triptans.*

Generic name	Dosage forms	Usual dosage
Sumatriptan	Tablets 25, 50, 100 mg	25–100 mg prn
	Spray 5, 20 mg	5–20 mg prn
	Injectable 6 mg sq	4–6 mg prn
Treximet	85 mg Sumatriptan/500 mg Naproxen	One tablet prn
Rizatriptan	Tablet 5, 10 mg	5–10 mg prn
Zolmitriptan	Tablets 2.5, 5 mg	2.5–5 mg prn
Almotriptan	Tablets 6.25, 12.5 mg	6.25, 12.5 mg prn
Eletriptan	Tablets 20, 40 mg	20, 40, mg prn

*For all triptans: use one dose at the onset of migraine; may take a second dose 2 hours later. No more than two doses in a day.

Table 3. Preventive therapies for pediatric migraine.

Drug	Dosage	Side effects
Propranolol	1-2 mg/kg/day	Fatigue, depression
Divalproex	10–25 mg/kg/day	Weight gain, hepatotoxicity, teratogenicity
Topiramate	1–2 mg/kg/day	Weight loss, kidney stones
Levetiracetam	20–40 mg/kg/day	Behavioral changes
Cyproheptadine	4–12 mg/day	Sedation, weight gain
Zonisamide	3–5 mg/kg/day	Sedation, behavioral changes
Amitriptyline	1 mg/kg/day	Sedation, cardiac effects

found on riverbanks in Germany. Doses generally used are 50 mg twice a day in the pediatric population, and 75 mg twice a day in the older adolescent or adult population. Side effects are minimal and include reflux and eructation. Also, good reproducible data are available for magnesium at doses of about 9 mg/kg per day both in pediatric and adult patients. It is generally well tolerated and may be especially helpful with menstrually related migraine; side effects are minimal. Limited data are available on riboflavin (400 mg/day), melatonin (3 mg/day), and also co-enzyme Q10.

A list of prescription medication for the prevention of migraine headaches is presented in Table 3. Toprimate is the most widely studied medication for the treatment of migraine in pediatric patients. Adolescents are usually prescribed 100–200 mg/day in one dose or divided into two doses. It was first approved as an anti-epilepsy medication, and side effects include anorexia, kidney stones, and possible cognitive difficulties (word retrieval problems). Doses used in adolescents are 100–200 mg/day divided twice a day.

Amitriptyline has also been used extensively and may be an excellent option for children and adolescents with sleep difficulties. Side effects can include weight gain, dry mouth and constipation. The US FDA has determined that this medication be used with caution in patients with depression secondary to increased risk for suicidal ideation.

The authors of several recent studies have established the safety and efficacy of divalproex in adolescent migraine prevention. Recommended doses are 10–25 mg/kg/day. It should be avoided in adolescent girls secondary to the risk of teratogenicity such as cardiac and neural tube defects. Other side effects include weight gain and hepatotoxicity.

Tension-Type Headaches

This type of headaches is probably the most common in both the pediatric and adult populations. They may be frequent episodic, from 1–14 headache days per month, or chronic, $\geq$ 15 headache days per month (Table 4). There are notable differences between tension and migraine headaches. The duration of the former is more variable, and the pain is generally less severe. The incidence of these headaches in the general pediatric population varies from 10% to 25%. Factors such as regular meals, adequate hydration, adequate amount of rest, and minimal caffeine consumption are important components of the treatment regimen. Adhering to a reasonable schedule and attaining a balance between work and leisure activities are equally important. Non-pharmacological therapies, such as biofeedback and relaxation therapy, may be helpful especially in children with concurrent psychological or behavior problems.

Abortive pharmacological therapies may include over-the-counter ibuprofen or acetaminophen. These are well tolerated, safe and do not require a prescription. There are but a few studies on preventive treatment for tension-type headaches. One of these is magnesium pidolate 2.25 g twice per day. Melatonin 3 mg/day has

Table 4. Frequent episodic tension-type headache.

Description:

Frequent episodes of headache lasting minutes to days. The pain is typically bilateral, pressing or tightening in quality and of mild to moderate intensity, and it does not worsen with routine physical activity. There is no nausea, but photophobia or phonophobia may be present.

Diagnostic criteria:

A. At least 10 episodes occurring on ≥ 1 but < 15 days per month for at least 3 months (≥ 12 and < 180 days per year) and fulfilling criteria B–D
B. Headache lasting from 30 minutes to 7 days
C. Headache has at least two of the following characteristics:
   1. bilateral location
   2. pressing/tightening (non-pulsating) quality
   3. mild or moderate intensity
   4. not aggravated by routine physical activity such as walking or climbing stairs
D. Both of the following:
   1. no nausea or emesis (anorexia may occur)
   2. no more than one of either photophobia or phonophobia
E. Not attributed to another disorder

also been used. A recent study employed this regimen in 22 patients with significant reduction in headache frequency, and it was generally well tolerated. Amitriptyline (a dose of 1 mg/kg/day) has also been used with good results and little side effects.

Chronic Daily Headaches

Either migraine or tension headaches may increase in frequency to near daily or everyday headaches satisfying ICHD-II criteria for chronic daily headache, ≥ 15 headache days per month on average for three months with headache duration of at least 4 hours. According to the World Health Organization, about 4% of adults and 2% of adolescents worldwide experience chronic daily headaches (CDH). In both children and adults, most have chronic migraine rather than chronic tension headache. Medication overuse headache (MOH) (analgesic use $\geq$ 3x/week for 3 months) occurs concomitantly in about 60% of adults, and 30–50% of adolescents with CDH.

Treatment of MOH starts with discontinuing the frequent use of analgesics. In a recent study, Kosoff *et al.* determined that this measure alone successfully reduces the number of headaches in patients with MOH. As for other headache syndromes, topiramate and amitriptyline have been shown to be effective in decreasing the severity of headaches.

References

Ahonen K, Hämäläinen ML, Hoppu EM. Nasal sumatriptan is effective in treatment of migraine attacks in children: a randomized trial. *Neurology.* 2004.62:883–887.

Ahonen K, Hämäläinen ML, Hoppu EM. A randomized trial of rizatriptan in migraine attacks in children. *Neurology.* 2006.67:1135–1140.

Anttila P. Tension-type headache in childhood and adolescence. *Lancet Neurol.* 2006.5: 268–274.

Apostol G, Cady RK, Laforet GA, *et al.* Divalproex extended-release in adolescent migraine prophylaxis: results of a randomized, double-blind, placebo-controlled study. *Headache.* 2008.48:1012–1025.

Bigal ME, Lipton RB, Tepper SJ, *et al.* Primary chronic daily headache and its subtypes in adolescents and adults. *Neurology.* 2004.63:843–847.

Headache Classification Subcommittee of the International Headache Society. The international classification of headache disorders, 2nd Edition. *Cephalalgia.* 2004.24 (Suppl 1).

Hershey AD, Powers SW, Bentti A, *et al.* Effectiveness of amitriptyline in the prophylactic management of childhood headaches. *Headache.* 2000.40:539–549.

Hershey AD, Powers SW, Vockell AL, et al. Coenzyme Q10 deficiency and response to supplementation in pediatric and adolescent migraine. *Headache.* 2007.47:73–80.

Kossoff EH, Mankad DN. Medication-overuse headache in children: is initial preventive therapy necessary? *J Child Neurol.* 2006.21:45–48.

Linder SL, Mathew NT, Cady RK, *et al.* Efficacy and tolerability of almotriptan in adolescents: a randomized, double-blind, placebo-controlled trial. *Headache.* 2008.48:1326–1336.

Lewis DW, Diamond S, Scott D, *et al.* Prophylactic treatment of pediatric migraine. *Headache.* 2004.44:230–237.

Lewis DW, Winner P, Hershey AD, *et al.* Efficacy of zolmitriptan nasal spray in adolescent migraine. *Pediatrics.* 2007.120:390–396.

Lewis D, Winner P, Saper J, *et al.* Randomized, double-blind, placebo-controlled study to evaluate the efficacy and safety of topiramate for migraine prevention in pediatric subjects 12 to 17 years of age. *Pediatrics.* 2009.23:924–934.

Miano S, Parisi P, Pelliccia A, *et al.* Melatonin to prevent migraine or tension-type headache in children. *Neurol Sci.* 2008.29:285–287.

Pakalnis A, Kring D. Zonisamide prophylaxis in refractory pediatric headache. *Headache.* 2006.46:804–807.

Pakalnis A, Kring D, Meier L. Levetiracetam prophylaxis in pediatric migraine — an open-label study. *Headache.* 2007.47:427–430.

Pakalnis A, Butz C, Splaingard D, *et al.* Emotional problems and prevalence of medication overuse in pediatric chronic daily headache. *J Child Neurol.* 2007.22:1356–1359.

Wang F, Van Den Eeden SK, Ackerson LM, *et al.* Oral magnesium oxide prophylaxis of frequent migrainous headache in children: a randomized, double-blind, placebo-controlled trial. *Headache.* 2003.43:601–610.

6

MANAGEMENT OF HEADACHES IN THE EMERGENCY DEPARTMENT

Rachel Smitek and Emile El-Shammaa

A 6-year-old male presents with his mother to the emergency department with the chief complaint of headache. The mother states the child has complained of head pain consistently for the past 3 days. The child is unable to describe the character of the pain. The mother states the child seems to complain more at night. Oral analgesics have provided some relief. The mother denies the child having had fever, nasal drainage, neck pain, cough, nausea, emesis, abdominal pain, rash, or trauma. The child has no significant past medical history and does not take any medications regularly. Vital signs are stable and the child is afebrile. Upon physical examination, a well-appearing child sits on his mother's lap. Sclera and conjunctiva are clear. The oropharynx is clear without erythema or exudates, and the child denies facial tenderness. There is no nasal drainage. Inspection of the right ear is normal. The left tympanic membrane is erythematous and bulging. The patient winces with tugging of the left ear. The child moves his neck without difficulty or evidence of pain. Cardiopulmonary and abdominal examination are benign. No rash is evident. Neurological examination reveals no focal deficit. Cranial nerves 2–12, sensation, and motor functions are intact. No gait abnormalities are evident. The child is diagnosed with acute otitis media.

Division of Emergency Medicine, Nationwide Children's Hospital and The Ohio State University, Columbus, Ohio, USA

He is sent home with a prescription for amoxicillin, instructed to continue oral analgesics for pain, and is to follow up with his primary care physician in 3–5 days.

Introduction

Headache is a frequent complaint in children and adolescents. The prevalence of headache has been reported to be as high as 80% in school-age and adolescent children. However, only 1.3% of pediatric emergency department visits are for the chief complaint of headache. Although this percentage is low, it can reasonably be deduced that this population may represent pre-selected patients who require a more thorough investigation of the etiology of the headache.

A common way of classifying headaches is either "primary" or "secondary." Primary headaches are usually self-limited. They are typically diagnosed based on symptoms and patterns of the headache. Primary headaches include migraine, tension headache, cluster headache, and chronic daily headache. Secondary headaches are those with identifiable etiologies. Such examples include infections (both viral and bacterial), carbon monoxide poisoning, increased intracranial pressure, and hypertensive encephalopathy. Most primary headaches are of benign etiology. It is the responsibility of the Emergency Department physician, however, to recognize life-threatening etiologies of headache. Presented in Table 1 are common primary and secondary causes of headaches in children.

In 1997, Burton *et al.* (1997) completed a study where they evaluated children who presented to a pediatric emergency department with the chief complaint of a headache. In this retrospective study, where data from 288 patients was analyzed, the authors reported the most common diagnosis assigned to these children was viral illness. The next most frequent diagnosis was sinusitis and migraine, respectively. Lewis and Qureshi (2000) reported similar findings. In their study, 57% of patients were diagnosed with an upper respiratory tract infection (URIs) as the cause of acute pediatric headache. Kan *et al.* (2000) found URIs constitute 88% of secondary non-neurological causes of headaches . These studies illustrate the benign nature of the majority of pediatric headaches seen in the emergency department.

In addition to primary and secondary, pediatric headaches can be grouped based on four temporal patterns: acute, acute recurrent, chronic progressive, and chronic non-progressive. Acute headaches are defined as a single episode of pain without prior events. They are most often caused by febrile illnesses, including sinusitis, pharyngitis, and otitis media, but can also be life-threatening, such as

Table 1. Primary and secondary causes of headache in children.

Primary

- Migraine
- Tension-type headache
- Cluster headache
- Chronic daily headaches

Secondary

- Infection
- Brain tumor
- Hydrocephalus
- Hypertension
- Pseudotumor cerebri
- Ventriculo-peritoneal shunt malfunction
- Malformations: Chiari
- Toxins: carbon monoxide, lead
- Post-lumbar puncture

Table 2. Pediatric acute headache etiologies.

- Febrile illness: URI, sinusitis, pharyngitis, otitis media
- Dental infection
- Trauma
- First episode of migraine
- CNS infections: meningitis, encephalitis, cerebral abscess
- Subarachnoid or intracranial hemorrhage
- Hydrocephalus
- VP shunt malfunction
- Toxins/substance abuse
- Carbon monoxide poisoning
- Hypertension
- Postictal

meningitis. Typically, children with more serious etiologies appear sicker. They may have a history of trauma or have worrisome findings on physical examination such as neck rigidity or lethargy. Children may have a history of neurosurgical interventions, such as having a ventriculo-peritoneal (VP) shunt which might have malfunctioned. Common etiologies for acute headache in children are listed in Table 2.

Acute recurrent headaches are episodes of head pain separated by symptom-free periods. The most common etiologies are migraine and tension-type headaches. Other causes include cluster headache, neuralgias, and headaches associated with epilepsy syndromes. Less than half of children with migraine headaches present with aura symptoms. These sensory symptoms typically occur within one hour of headache onset and are usually visual. Migraines in children are typically bilateral and can last 1–72 hours. Children can present with nausea, emesis, anorexia, irritability, or malaise.

Chronic progressive headaches are the most worrisome. These gradually increase in frequency and intensity over time. Brain tumors are of significant concern when parents present to the emergency department with their child who has been complaining of a headache. Typically, headaches associated with brain tumors are those that occur late at night or early in the morning and have worsened over time. The headache can awaken the child from sleep. Night-time or early morning emesis can be a sign of increased intracranial pressure, causing the child's headache. In addition, the child may experience a change in behavior, mood, or school performance. Lewis and Qureshi (2000) reported that pediatric patients with acute onset headache and who were eventually diagnosed with a brain tumor or intracranial hemorrhages had neurological abnormalities. These included papilledema, ataxia, or abnormal eye movements. Joseph and Webb (2005) found there are five key elements to the neurological exam that need to be assessed and documented when brain tumor is a concern: optic discs, eye movements, pronator drift, tandem gait, and deep tendon reflexes.

A second common cause of chronic progressive headaches is idiopathic intracranial hypertension (IIH) or pseudotumor cerebri. The condition is defined by three criteria: papilledema, increased intracranial pressure with normal CSF chemistry, and normal brain imaging. The headaches are caused by persistently increased intracranial pressure, likely due to impaired resorption of CSF by the arachnoid villi. IIH has been linked to obesity, use of birth control pills, head trauma, otitis media, and excessive vitamin A intake. Symptoms of IIH include emesis, neck pain, ataxia, and blurred vision (for a detailed discussion on IIH, see Chapter 16). Common causes of chronic progressive pediatric headaches are listed in Table 3.

Chronic non-progressive headaches are defined as 15 or more headaches a month for 4 or more months. These headaches usually last 4 or more hours. Emotional and psychological worries are common causes which explain the normal neurological examination.

Another cause of chronic non-progressive cephalea in children is post-traumatic headache. These headaches can occur up to 8 weeks after the injury.

Table 3. Common causes of chronic progressive headaches in children.

- Brain tumor
- Idiopathic intracranial hypertension
- Hydrocephalus
- Infection: chronic meningitis due to fungi, tuberculosis, and neuroborreliosis
- Hypertension
- Malformations
- Subdural hematoma
- Vascular malformations

Children often complain of dizziness. Post-traumatic headaches can have features similar to both migraines and tension type headaches.

It is estimated that 6.6% to 6.9% of pediatric headaches are due to a serious neurological condition. Among these are brain tumors, viral meningitis, intracranial hemorrhage, and VP shunt malfunction. The most common serious neurological condition is viral meningitis.

The headache of a serious neurological disease usually presents with pain that has been present for less than 2 months . Both location and quality of the pain have been shown to be valuable information in the assessment of serious versus non–life-threatening headache. Conicella *et al.* (2008) found that over 70% of primary headaches were unilateral. In contrast, patients who were either unable to locate the pain or who indicated the pain was occipital were found to have serious underlying illness. All patients with primary headaches were able to describe the quality of the pain (constrictive, pulsating, stabbing etc.). Conversely, 8.3% to 50% of children with serious underlying illness were unable to describe the quality of pain. These findings support the notion that a thorough history and physical examination are paramount in identifying potentially serious etiologies.

Clinical Approach To Evaluating A Child With The Chief Complaint Of Headache

As indicated above, most headache syndromes can be diagnosed based on clinical history. First, the characteristics of the headache should be explored. Information regarding the mode of onset (abrupt vs. gradual), timing (morning vs. evening), and frequency of headaches can aid in identifying a cause. For example, a headache that awakens a child from sleep may represent a brain tumor. Additionally, an abrupt onset of a painful headache may signify an intracranial hemorrhage. Next, questions concerning the duration, location, quality and severity of pain should

Table 4. Assessment of pediatric headache.

- Mode of onset: An abrupt painful headache may represent an intracranial hemorrhage.
- Timing: Tension headache typically occurs late in the day. In contrast, a headache that awakens a child from sleep is concerning for a brain tumor.
- Frequency: Acute, recurrent headaches are typically primary headaches, such as a migraine. A chronic, progressive headache may represent a mass lesion (such as tumor, abscess, or hemorrhage).
- Duration: Migraine headaches can last up to 72 hours.
- Location: Infection-related headaches (such as sinusitis) and migraines are usually unilateral. Occipital headaches should raise the suspicion for a more worrisome etiology (such as tumor).
- Quality/severity of pain: Children with upper respiratory infections are likely able to describe the type of pain, in contrast to those with serious underlying illness.

be asked in order to arrive at an accurate diagnosis. These questions are listed on Table 4.

Information on exacerbating and relieving factors, treatments, pain compared to prior headaches, and history of trauma are all important in evaluating the current pain crisis. Furthermore, symptoms associated with a headache can clue a clinician in on the correct diagnosis. Burton *et al.* (1997) found the majority of children with viral meningitis were likely to present with fever (73%), emesis (73%), and neck pain (53%) in addition to the chief complaint of a headache. Acute exposure to carbon monoxide in children is likely to render symptoms similar to those of influenza or gastroenteritis. Additionally, other household members may present with similar symptoms suggesting carbon monoxide exposure. Migraines can be associated with or without a visual aura in addition to nausea, emesis, photophobia, and phonophobia. Finally, questions about medication and toxin exposure, pre-existing medical conditions, and family history need to be asked. Family history is particularly important in such conditions as migraines and carbon monoxide exposure. Examples of clinical history questions are listed in Table 5.

Which Physical Examination Findings Are Helpful In Reaching A Diagnosis?

A thorough physical examination should follow the clinical history. Vital signs and general appearance can be the first indicators of a sick child. Fever is a common finding in children with headaches due to viral meningitis. Headache in the presence of a rash can indicate bacterial meningitis. Elevated blood pressure

Table 5. Clinical history of headaches in children and adolescents.

- When did your headache start?
- What were you doing when the headache began?
- Have you had headaches like this in the past? How is this headache different?
- Where does your head hurt? Describe your headache.
- How long do your headaches last? How often do your headaches occur?
- What makes your headache better? What makes it feel worse?
- What type of symptoms do you have with your headache (nausea, emesis, vision changes, numbness, weakness, or other symptoms)?
- Does anyone else in your family have headaches?
- What other medical problems do you have?
- What medications do you take?
- Why did this headache cause you to seek medical attention?
- What do you think is causing your headache?

can be the cause of a headache or a marker of intracranial pathology. A head and neck examination may reveal signs of facial tenderness as seen in sinusitis, dental injury, or infection. Pharyngeal exudates may be suggestive of *Streptococcal pharyngitis.* Nuchal rigidity is present in 63% of children with viral meningitis. Most children with headaches will have a normal neurological examination. In fact, the authors of one study showed that all children with migraine or URI-related headaches have normal neurological examinations. While a normal neurological examination may be reassuring, focal findings are highly suggestive of serious underlying illness. One should assess the child's mental status if possible. Altered mental status can represent hypoxia, hypoglycemia, toxin exposure, seizure, or intracranial pathology. As part of the fundoscopic examination, the physician should look for papilledema that may be associated with increased intracranial pressure, or hemorrhages which may signify trauma or intracranial hemorrhage. The cranial nerves examination can help locate a mass lesion. Asymmetry or weakness in the motor or sensory examination can suggest a focal lesion. Finally, abnormalities in coordination, deep tendon reflexes, gait, and a positive Romberg sign may aid in the final diagnosis of a cerebellar disorder. While focal abnormalities in the neurological examination may be red flags for a serious underlying disease, it is important to realize that absence of these signs does not eliminate the possibility of serious pathology.

The utility of laboratory tests depends on the suspected etiology of the headache. A rapid strep antigen test is useful in a child with sore throat, fever, and headache. A bedside glucose test can uncover hypoglycemia as the source of the headache. Most children presenting with a headache to the emergency department do not require laboratory testing. However, if a serious etiology is suspected, the work-up should reflect the differential diagnosis. Complete blood count, blood cultures, and cerebrospinal fluid analysis are indicated if there is concern for an infectious process. Lumbar puncture is typically employed in cases where infection (meningitis, encephalitis), subarachnoid hemorrhage, and idiopathic intracranial hypertension are high on the list of possible diagnoses. In cases of suspected infection, the CSF should be tested for the presence of cells, protein and glucose content, Gram stain, and CSF bacterial cultures. The CSF's opening pressure should always be measured. CT scan of the head needs to be done prior to the LP in children suspected to have a subarachnoid hemorrhage or elevated intracranial pressure. Additional studies that may be helpful in the evaluation include: coagulation studies, carboxyhemoglobin levels, lead levels, toxicology screen, thyroid function studies, serum electrolytes, urine analysis, urine pregnancy test, and ECG. It is important to remember these tests are used to aid in the diagnostic process, rather than to make the diagnosis.

The majority of children with headaches do not require radiological evaluation. Lateef *et al.* (2009) studied 364 children ages 2–5 years of age who presented to a pediatric ED with the chief complaint of headache to determine whether computed tomography of the head led to better care. They found that, based on history and physical examination, 306 children had an identifiable cause for their headache. Of those, 57 children had undergone head CT, eight of which had an abnormal scan. While the reason for ordering the test was not outlined, final diagnoses for causes of secondary headaches included: trauma, seizure, VP shunt failure, brain tumor, stroke, meningitis, and non-neurologic causes. The authors of the study concluded that for children presenting with headache, non-worrying history, and a normal neurological examination, the head CT did not add much to the evaluation.

A head CT should be considered in children suspected of having an intracranial lesion or hemorrhage (Figures 1–4). Children with serious neurological conditions with worrisome histories or abnormalities on physical examination warrant undergoing a scan. Furthermore, children with worsening chronic progressive headaches, abrupt onset, or significant risk factors such as trauma or presence of a VP shunt may need a CT scan (Figures 5–6). These indications are listed in Table 6.

Headache treatment

Since the majority of headaches are benign, reassurance is an important aspect of the management. The treatment should be directed towards the cause of the child's headache. Often, the use of oral analgesics is an effective therapy. In cases involving an infectious etiology, antibiotics are indicated. Patients may need further

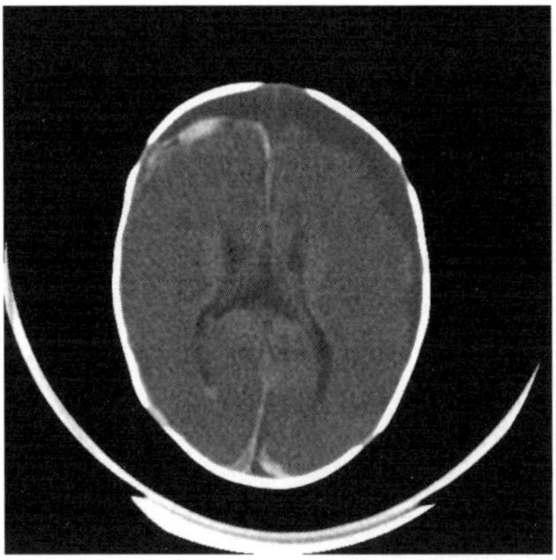

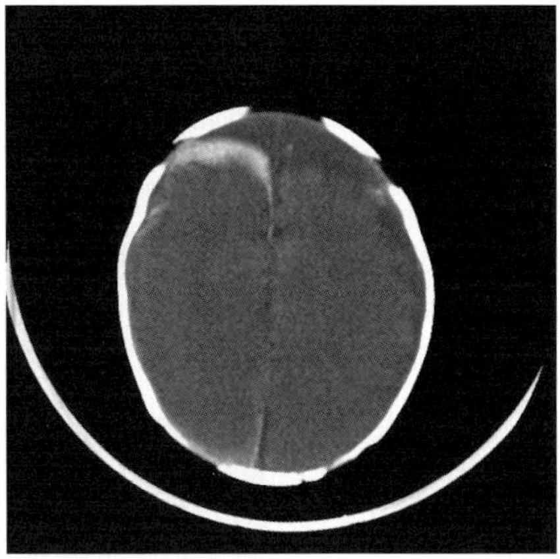

Figures 1–2. Bilateral acute and chronic subdural hematoma in an abused child.

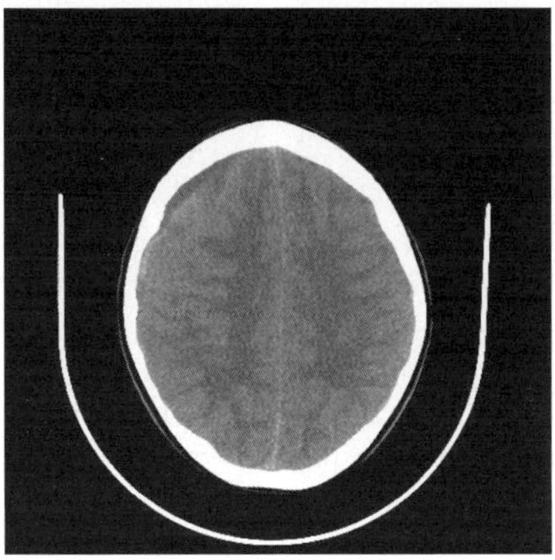

Figure 3. Chronic subdural hematoma.

evaluation by a neurosurgeon if VP shunt malfunction is diagnosed. Presented in Figure 7 is a flowchart which helps guide the assessment and management of various acute pediatric headache syndromes.

Migraine

For acute recurrent headaches such as migraines, ibuprofen (10 mg/kg) and acetaminophen (15 mg/kg) are considered first line. Ketorolac is a good option when the patient is experiencing nausea and emesis. In addition to analgesics,

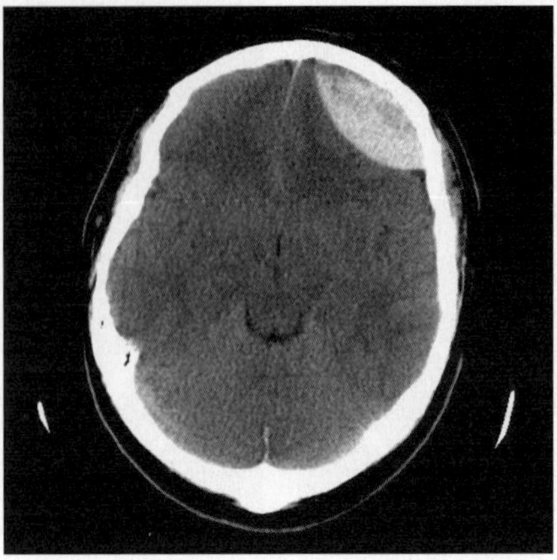

Figure 4. Epidural hematoma.

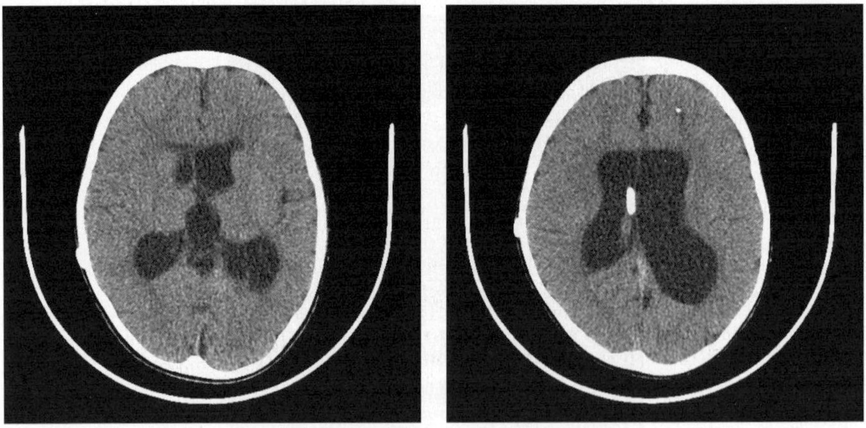

Figures 5–6. VP shunt failure with acute hydrocephalus.

Table 6. Indications for head CT.

- Concerning history: prior neurosurgical intervention, pain upon awakening
- Concerning physical examination findings: papilledema, ataxia, hemiparesis, abnormal eye movements, depressed deep tendon reflexes
- Worsening chronic, progressive headache
- Abrupt onset of headache
- Risk factors: trauma, VP shunt

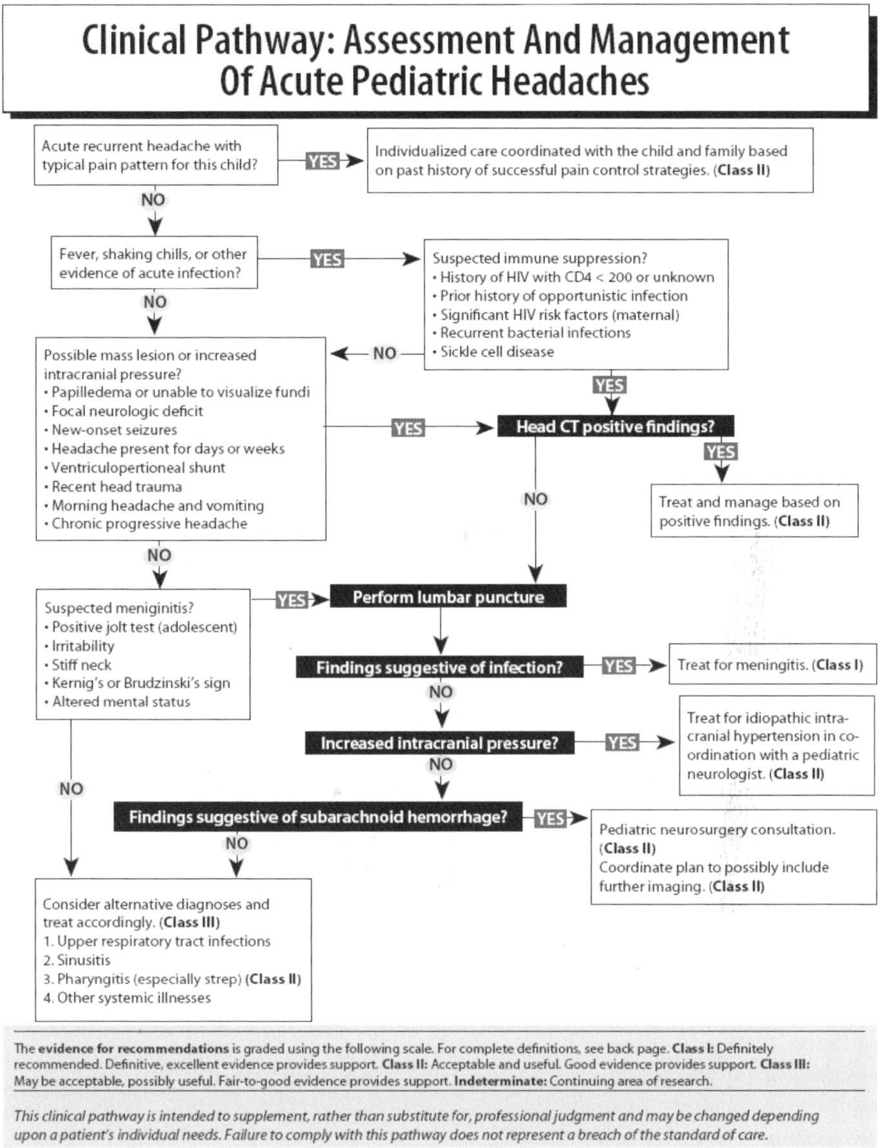

Figure 7. Assessment and management of acute pediatric headaches. Joseph MM, Webb K. Evidence-based assessment and treatment of acute headache in children and adolescents in the ED. *Pediatric Emergency Medicine Practice.* 2005;2(5):14. www.ebmedicine.net

antiemetics are useful in the treatment of migraines. Metoclopramide, prochlorperazine, and promethazine are dopamine antagonists that have been proven to provide headache relief in addition to having antiemetic properties. While antiemetics are useful, they are not without side effects including dystonia and tardive dyskinesia. Triptans are also effective for acute migraine headache relief. These agents are serotonin-receptor agonists that act as cerebral vasoconstrictions. The authors of several studies have shown that sumatriptan nasal spray is effective in children (5 mg) and adolescents (20 mg) with migraines. However, there is not enough data to support the use of any oral triptan or subcutaneous sumatriptan. Bad taste is the most common side effect of the nasal spray. The treatment approach to a child with acute onset migraine headache presenting to the emergency department should start with simple oral analgesics, either ibuprofen or acetaminophen, and rest in a quiet room. If the child complains of nausea and emesis, the use of an antiemetic plus the need for intravenous fluids should be assessed. If the child still complains of pain, nasal sumatriptan should be considered. The use of narcotics should be a measure of last resort for the treatment of acute migraine headaches in children and adolescents. Migraine prophylaxis is best managed by the child's primary care physician or possibly a neurologist. Therapies need to be individualized, requiring adherence by the patient.

Cluster headache

Acute onset cluster headaches are treated like migraines. Subcutaneous sumatriptan and 100% O_2 at a rate of 8–10 L/min have been shown to be effective.

Tension headaches

Like migraines and cluster headaches, oral analgesics are effective for the treatment of tension headaches. Since tension headaches are typically triggered by stressful events, recognizing what these triggers are and subsequently modifying lifestyle choices may provide relief. Counseling and biofeedback techniques may aid recognizing stressors.

Pseudotumor cerebri

Children may require hospitalization if the symptoms are severe or persistent. However, the physician can remove sufficient CSF to reduce the pressure to less than 20-cm H_2O. Acetazolamide (Diamox) decreases CSF production and can be started in the emergency department. Optimally, a neurologist and ophthalmologist should be involved in the patient's care. Please see Chapter 16 on IIH.

Posttraumatic headaches

These headaches are usually due to stress and anxiety, and typically resolve within 3–6 months. Simple analgesics and non-pharmacological therapies, such as biofeedback and relaxation techniques, can be helpful. In some instances, antidepressants or anticonvulsants are used.

Patient resources

Parents and teenagers can learn about headaches by visiting the website of the American Academy of Pediatrics (http://www.aap.org). This resource outlines several headache types that teens may experience. Additionally, the website lists signs and symptoms that may warrant seeking evaluation by a healthcare professional.

The American Academy of Neurology also offers patient information regarding headaches. In addition to providing general information, the website (http://patients.aan.com/go/home) lists various resources and contact information that may benefit certain patient populations.

Acknowledgements

Special thanks to Lisa C. Martin, MD, Children's Radiological Institute at Nationwide Children's Hospital, for her generous contribution of the images for this article.

References

Burton LJ, Quinn B, *et al.* Headache etiology in a pediatric emergency department. *Pediatr Emerg Care.* 1997.13:1–4.

Conicella E, Raucci U, Vanacore N, *et al.* The child with headache in a pediatric ED. *Headache.* 2008.48:1005–1011.

Joseph MM, Webb K. Evidence-based assessment and treatment of acute headache in children and adolescents in the ED. *Ped Emerg Med Pract.* 2005.2:1–28.

Kan L, Nagelberg J, Maytal J. Headaches in a pediatric emergency department: etiology, imaging, and treatment. *Headache.* 2000.40:25–29.

King C. Emergent evaluation of headache in children. www.uptodate.com. 2009.1–22.

Lateef TM, Grewal M, *et al.* Headache in young children in the emergency department: use of computed tomography. *Pediatrics.* 2009.124:e12–e17.

Lewis DW, Qureshi F. Acute headache in children and adolescents presenting to the emergency department. *Headache.* 2000.40:200–203.

Qureshi F, Lewis D. Managing headache in the pediatric emergency department. *Clin Ped Emerg Med.* 2003.4:159–170.

7

AUTISM SPECTRUM DISORDERS

Emily de los Reyes

A 20-month-old male is brought for evaluation by his parents because they are concerned he may have language delay. The boy just recently started to walk but still tends to fall. The child enjoys watching television and puts his face up close to the television screen. The boy does not have spoken language, nor does he like to point at objects. He, however, likes to hum. The youngster prefers to line up blocks and likes to spin the wheels of cars. His physical and neurological examinations are normal except for low muscle tone. The child makes poor eye contact and tends to flap his hands; he has no dysmorphic features.

The boy in the vignette exhibits repetitive behavior (hand flapping and visual inspection), delayed language (no intelligible speech), and poor social communication (poor eye contact and no gestures). For those reasons, it is highly suspicious that the child has a neurodevelopmental disorder such as autism. Current recommendations by the American Academy of Pediatrics is that a child with the above mentioned signs and symptoms undergo an evaluation to determine if the child has autism.

Introduction

Autism spectrum disorders are a group of conditions that encompass deficits in language, poor social skills, and stereotypic behaviors. The diagnostic criteria for autism is detailed in the Diagnostic and Statistical Manual of Mental Disorders,

Division of Child Neurology, Nationwide Children's Hospital and The Ohio State University, Columbus, Ohio, USA

Fourth edition (DSM-IV) (Table 1). The prevalence of autism is 6 per 1000. This number has increased in the current millennium most likely because of increased awareness and broadened criteria to include children with Asperger syndrome and pervasive developmental disorders not otherwise specified.

Autism is a neurodevelopment disorder characterized by deficits in communication, socialization, and by the presence of repetitive and stereotypic behaviors. The language disorder is characterized by delay in the development of spoken language or difficulties sustaining conversational speech. Echolalia and idiosyncratic speech are also hallmarks of the condition. Patients with autism exhibit a social disorder characterized by marked impairment in the use of nonverbal cues such as gestures and poor eye contact. Patients with autism also exhibit deficits in socialization with peers such as difficulty initiating and sustaining peer-play and interaction. Repetitive patterns of behavior like finger and hand flapping, and twisting or complex body movements are common in these patients. The parents of children who may eventually be diagnosed as having autism usually voice their concerns to the child's primary care physician by 15 to 18 months of age. Some children however, are not diagnosed until much later.

Diagnosis

Early identification of the disorder is essential as this allows implementation of specific interventions to improve patient outcomes. The diagnosis of autism is made on clinical grounds. That said, several genetic disorders are associated with autism spectrum disorders. A thorough physical and neurological exam is essential to tailor therapeutic recommendations to each child. The presence of dysmorphic features and focal deficits on the neurological exam may provide clues to the etiology of the condition. These might include Rett syndrome, Angelman syndrome, fragile-X and tuberous sclerosis complex. Genetic microarray testing may help detect microdeletions, microduplications, and subtelomeric or unbalanced chromosomal rearrangements. *De novo* microdeletion and microduplication of chromosome 16p11.2 was recently found in 1% of patients with autism. Other chromosomal abnormalities associated with autism include chromosome 15 duplication. Rarely, a metabolic disorder may be considered in children with autism, especially if regression is identified. It is important to identify this subgroup of patients because they are at higher risk for autistic regression which may present with loss of language skills, epilepsy, hypotonia, or poor growth. Adequate hydration, fever-control, and enzyme replacement may be essential for this subgroup of patients. Radiological evaluation is not necessary for the diagnosis of autism unless there is a co-morbid disorder like microcephaly, epilepsy or mental retardation.

Table 1. Diagnostic and statistical manual of mental disorders.

1. Diagnostic Criteria for 299.00: AD

A. A total of six (or more) items from (1), (2), and (3), with at least two from (1), and one each from (2) and (3):

(1) Qualitative impairment in social interaction, as manifested by at least two of the following:

  (a) Marked impairment in the use of multiple nonverbal behaviors such as eye-to-eye gaze, facial expression, body postures, and gestures to regulate social interaction.
  (b) Failure to develop peer relationships appropriate to developmental level.
  (c) A lack of spontaneous seeking to share enjoyment, interests, or achievements with other people (e.g., by a lack of showing, bringing, or pointing out objects of interest).
  (d) Lack of social or emotional reciprocity.

(2) Qualitative impairments in communication as manifested by at least one of the following:

  (a) Delay in or total lack of, the development of spoken language (not accompanied by an attempt to compensate through alternative modes of communication such as gesture of mine).
  (b) In individuals with adequate speech, marked impairment in the ability to initiate or sustain a conversation with others.
  (c) Stereotyped and repetitive use of language or idiosyncratic language.
  (d) Lack of varied, spontaneous make-believe play or social imitative play appropriate to developmental level.

(3) Restricted repetitive and stereotyped patterns of behavior, interests, and activities as manifested by at least one of the following:

  (a) Encompassing preoccupation with one or more stereotyped and restricted patterns of interest that is abnormal either in intensity or focus.
  (b) Apparently inflexible adherence to specific, nonfunctional routines or rituals
  (c) Stereotyped and repetitive motor mannerisms (e.g., hand or finger flapping or twisting, or complex whole-body movements).
  (d) Persistent preoccupation with parts of objects.

B. Delays or abnormal functioning in at least one of the following areas, with onset before 3 years old: (1) social interaction, (2) language as used in social communication, or (3) symbolic or imaginative play.

C. The disturbance is not better accounted for by Rett's Disorder or childhood disintegrative disorder.

Reprinted with permission from American Psychiatric Association. Diagnostic and Statistical Manual of Mental Disorders, Fourth Edition, Text Revision (DSM-IV-TR). Washington, DC, USA.

Psychological Testing

The Modified Checklist for Autism in Toddlers (MCHAT) is an easy-to-use tool. However, it may be less sensitive for the identification of patients with milder variants of autism, those without mental retardation or older children. The most commonly used tools for the diagnosis of autism include the Childhood Autism Rating Scales (trained observer), Gilliam Autism Rating Scale (parental report), and Autism Diagnostic Observation Schedule revised (ADOS). The ADOS is a semi-structured, play-based assessment of communication and social skills. Other autism-specific diagnostic measures include the Pervasive Developmental Disorders Behavior Inventory (PDDBI) which is a parent report that assesses autistic behaviors. It is also important that the child's cognitive abilities be measured using age-appropriate tools. This information assists in program planning for school and therapies. Language abilities are assessed by the speech-language therapist using the Preschool Language Scales (PLS-4). It is also recommended that all children undergo a formal audiological evaluation.

Co-Morbid Disorders

Several conditions are commonly associated with autism. These include attention deficit disorder, mental retardation, and epilepsy.

Mental retardation

Mental retardation is defined as "significantly sub-average general intellectual functioning with an intelligence quotient score (IQ) of < 70, existing concurrently with deficits in adaptive behavior and manifested during the developmental period, which adversely affects a child's educational performance." Mild mental retardation is associated with an IQ of 50–70 with an incidence of 20–30/1000. Severe mental retardation is associated with an IQ of less than 50 and has an incidence of 3–4/1000. Tests used to evaluate a child's mental capabilities include: the Stanford Binet Intelligence Scales 5th ed. (SB5), Wechsler Intelligence Scales for children, Wechsler Individual Achievement tests and, Mullen Scales of Early Learning and Wide Range Achievement Test. Deficits in adaptive behavior is documented using Vineland scales.

Epilepsy

The incidence of epilepsy in children with autism is as high as 50%. Although not all children have clinical manifestations, it is important to consider Landau-Kleffner syndrome. This is especially important for children who have autistic regression or if the child presents with sudden loss of language. Treatment depends on the clinical manifestations and the classification of the epileptic syndrome. Oftentimes, the clinician may choose a medication which has a positive impact on both behavior and attention problems as these tend to co-exist in children with autism.

Treatment

The management of autism is based on the principles of behavioral and educational intervention. It is also recommended that referral to a local early intervention program be made as soon as the diagnosis is confirmed.

Applied behavioral analysis (ABA) is the process of applying interventions based on the principles of learning. These are derived from experimental psychology research. The aim is to systematically change a behavior and demonstrate that the interventions used are responsible for the observed improvement. ABA methods are used to increase and maintain desirable adaptive behaviors, reduce interfering maladaptive behaviors or limit the conditions under which they occur, teach new skills, and generalize behaviors to new environments or situations. Another program that is well accepted is structured teaching or the TEACCH (Treatment and Education of Autistic or Communication-related Handicapped Children). The principles of this program emphasize structure and organization. Other interventions include speech and language therapy, and occupational therapy.

Speech therapy is an invaluable tool in the management of children with autism spectrum disorders. However, alternative and augmentive communication methods are also recommended, especially if the child fails to develop spoken language. The Picture Exchange System (PECS) allows children to communicate their needs through the use of pictographs. As children mature and cognition improves, the use of more sophisticated augmentive communication methods is recommended.

Pharmacological treatment for autism's co-morbid disorders includes the use of narcoleptics, antipsychotics, and selective serotonin reuptake inhibitors. There is evidence to support the use of risperidone to treat impaired social behavior, interfering repetitive phenomena, and aggression. Selective serotonin reuptake inhibitors are used for the treatment of conditions such as depression, anxiety, and obsessive-compulsive behaviours.

Asperger Syndrome

Asperger syndrome (AS) is a neurodevelopmental disorder characterized by deficits in social interactions, and the presence of pragmatic language and restricted interests. Children with Asperger syndrome have normal acquisition of language skills and average cognitive skills. Children with AS are diagnosed at an older age than those with autism; the average age of diagnosis is 6 years. This is most likely a reflection of the increasing social demands of school which lead to the evaluation of the child's atypical behaviours. The language deficits of children with AS may include difficulties in non-literal idiomatic speech including poor understanding of humor, sarcasm, or figures of speech. Prosody may be monotonous and their language has been characterized as "pedantic."

Pervasive Developmental Disorders

Pervasive developmental disorder is a term used to include children with impairments in social, language, or behavior skills, but on a milder degree than those with AS.

Attention Deficit Disorder

Attention deficit disorder (ADD) is one of the most common neuropsychiatric disorders. The condition may become evident at any time during the child's life. That said, it is most commonly diagnosed during the school years. Of late, there has been increased awareness of the condition in young adults. The core symptoms of ADD are hyperactivity, and deficits of attention and vigilance. The Diagnostic and Statistical Manual IV requires the presence of six out of the nine symptoms in the inattention cluster and the hyperactivity cluster. Symptoms included in the inattention cluster are: inattention, poor organization, forgetfulness, and failing to give attention to details. Symptoms within the hyperactive cluster include: talking excessively, blurting out answers, frequent interruptions, and verbal intrusions. A thorough history and physical examination are necessary. The case history should include birth, developmental, and social history, as well as that of any associated medical condition. Children may be identified during the school age, secondary to them exhibiting learning disorders or behavior problems. The most commonly used behavior rating scales include: Connor's parent and teacher rating scales, childhood behavior check list, and Vanderbilt ADHD parents and teacher questionnaire. Radiological evaluation of a patient with ADD or ADHD is not indicated. An electroencephalogram may be necessary if the history is consistent with seizures, especially absence epilepsy.

Treatment

The medications most commonly recommended for the treatment of attention deficit disorder are stimulants; specifically, methylphenidate and amphetamine.

Fifteen to thirty percent of children who take medication for ADHD experience transient tics. In addition to pharmacotherapy, children with ADD benefit from what are called "school modifications." These include: small class size, preferential classroom seating, and assistance organizing their work.

References

American Psychiatric Association. *Diagnostic and Statistical Manual of Mental Disorders.* 4th ed. 1994. Washington DC. International Classification of Diseases: Diagnostic Criteria for Research, 10th ed., by the World Health Organization.

CDC. *Surveillance Summaries.* MMWE Morbid Mortal Wkly Rep. 2007.56:1–28.

Filipek PA, Accardo PJ, Ashwal G, *et al.* Practice parameter: screening and diagnosis of autism: report of the Quality Standards Subcommittee of the American Academy of Neurology and the Child Neurology Society. *Neurology.* 2000.55:468–479.

Johnson CP, Myers SM and Council on Children with Disabilities. Identification and Evaluation of Children with autism spectrum disorders. *Pediatrics.* 2007.120:1182–1215.

Levy SE, Hyma SL and Pinto-Martin J. Autism spectrum disorders. In: Accardo PJ, (ed.) *Neurodevelopmental Disabilities in Infancy and Childhood. Vol. 2.* 3rd ed. Baltimore, MD: Brookes Publishing. 2008. pp. 497.

Shen Y, Dries KA, Holm IA, *et al.* Clinical genetic testing for patients with Autistic spectrum disorders. *Pediatrics.* 2010.125:e727–e735.

Sebat J, Lakshmi B, Malhotra D, *et al.* Strong association of de novo copy number mutations in autism. *Science.* 2007.316:445–449.

Shoffner J, Hams L, Langley G, *et al.* Fever plus Mitochondrial disease could be risk factors for autistic regression. *J Child Neurol.* 2010.25:429–434.

Pliska S and AACAP Work Group on Quality issues. Practice parameter for the assessment and treatment of children and adolescents with attention-deficit/hyperactivity disorder. *J Am Acad Child Adolesc Psychiatry.* 2007.46:894–921.

Weiss LA, Shen Y, Korn JM, *et al.* Association between microdeletion and microduplication at 16p 11.2 and autism. *N Engl J Med.* 2008.358:667–675.

8

NEURODEVELOPMENTAL DISORDERS

Emily de los Reyes

A 15-year-old boy with a diagnosis of "sensory processing disorder" and language delay is seen in the office for an initial evaluation. The boy has an elongated triangular face and prominent ears. The boy receives special education services at school. The family has requested a neurological evaluation because of the young man's worsening behavior.

Introduction

The evaluation of a patient with the diagnosis of developmental disorder can be quite daunting. Commonly, families indicate that their child has failed to acquire major developmental milestones. The use of comparative genomic hybridization techniques and magnetic resonance imaging has facilitated the identification of specific disorders in children with developmental delay. In this chapter, I discuss the evaluation of the child with such conditions.

Clinical history

As part of the evaluation of a child with a neurodevelopmental disorder, there are certain key points that a clinician should carefully consider. Developmental delay may be global (speech, motor, and social) or restricted to a specific domain. Considering this difference provides clues for certain diagnoses, which may help

Division of Child Neurology, Nationwide Children's Hospital and The Ohio State University, Columbus, Ohio, USA

guide the clinician toward specific interventions. It is also important to determine whether the delay is static or progressive. It is imperative to ask the parents whether there has been loss of previously acquired skills as is seen in patients with progressive neurodegenerative and metabolic diseases. Otherwise, most disorders are static or have a slow and steady improvement.

As part of the case history, the clinician needs to gather information on risk factors that may result in developmental delay. The prenatal history may provide clues to the timing of the insult. It is important to obtain details about previous pregnancies as well as that of the child being evaluated. This information includes: recurrent miscarriages, maternal infections, exposure to substances of abuse or alcohol, exposure to medications, prenatal bleeding, premature labor, stillbirths, obstetrical complications, premature birth, low birth-weight, and multi-fetus pregnancies. For instance, a history of recurrent miscarriages may be a clue for genetic or metabolic inherited diseases. An infant with low birth-weight may be at risk for intraventricular hemorrhage, sepsis, meningitis, metabolic derangements, and nutritional deficits which may have impacted the growth of the brain. Patients with predominately motor impairment, a history of prematurity or a history of perinatal complications, are at risk for periventricular leukomalacia. In those instances, radiological evaluation of the brain, ideally using MRI, may help identify the cause of the impairment. This information can then be used for the purposes of prognosis and management. Information on perinatal adverse events such as premature birth, hypoxic-ischemic insult, seizures, multi-organ failure, infections, or intraventricular hemorrhage may help arrive at a diagnosis. For details on these, see Chapter 20.

As would be expected, significant information can be drawn from the child's family medical history. Special attention needs to be placed on the presence of mental retardation, learning disabilities, or developmental delay in the parents or extended family. It is important to inquire about parental consanguinity as well as a family history of deafness, blindness or chromosomal abnormalities. From a psycho-social standpoint, it is important that the clinician inquire about stressful life events — divorce, death, unemployment — which can trigger depression and other psychopathology. It is well known that, in those circumstances, parents may neglect their children and hence cause delayed development or learning disabilities. Children who live below the poverty level are also at risk for illiteracy and suboptimal health.

Physical examination

Information derived from the physical examination is as important as that from the clinical history. Head circumference growth is a parameter that may point to a potential cause of the child's delayed development. For example, microcephaly detected at the time of the child's birth may indicate that the newborn has endured *in utero* infection with one of the TORCH pathogens. Evaluation of the skin may reveal the presents of lesions such as *café-au-lait* spots as seen in patients with neurofibromatosis. Hepatosplenomegaly may be seen in patients with a storage disease or metabolic derangements. Finally, neurological signs such as decrease in the level of awareness, hypotonia, spasticity, abnormal reflexes, or focal cranial nerve finding may be seen in children with neurodevelopmental disorders.

Neurogenetics

The field of neurogenetics has been revolutionized by the successful sequencing of the human genome. The technique of array comparative genomic hybridization (CGH) allows for high-resolution, genome-wide screening of segmental genomic copy number variations. It also helps detect deletions, duplications, and chromosome gains and losses. CGH, however, does not help detect balanced rearrangements and genetic alterations (uniparental disomy, imprinting and other epigenetic alterations). Current recommendations from the American College of Medical Genetics, is that CGH testing be carried out in children with developmental delay, multiple congenital abnormalities, and autism spectrum disorders. The differential diagnosis of developmental delay is extensive and hence, testing should be tailored to the history and physical exam.

Trisomy 21 (Down syndrome) is the most common cause of developmental delay secondary to a chromosomal abnormality. The condition accounts for approximately 20% of all patients with developmental delay. Patients with Trisomy 21 need to undergo yearly evaluations. Areas of concerns include cognitive decline, early onset of Alzheimer-type dementia, obstructive sleep apnea, cardiac arrest, and cervical spine instability.

Fragile X syndrome is the next most common cause of mental retardation in children. The condition is caused by an expanded CGG triplet repeat in the first exon of the long arm of the Fragile X mental retardation gene (FMR1). Premutation carriers may have repeat expansions between 50 and 200 repeats. Fragile X syndrome manifests itself in individuals who have more than 200 CGG repeats. Symptomatic females have a milder degree of mental retardation than males. Children with Fragile X syndrome have dysmorphic features including macrocephaly and a long narrow face with prominent ears. They also have pre-pubertal macro-orchidism and excessive joint laxity. These individual may have mental retardation and exhibit hyperactivity. They may also have autistic features.

Some premutation carriers may develop ataxia and tremors as well as cognitive dysfunction in adulthood, mimicking parkinsonism.

Angelman syndrome is more commonly known as the "happy puppet" syndrome. Patients with Angelman syndrome have mental retardation, developmental delay, hypotonia, ataxia, mixed expressive-receptive language delay, paroxysmal and out of context laughter, and seizures. The most common genetic defect leading to Angelman syndrome is maternal deletion of a 4Mb region in the chromosomal region 15q11-q13 causing UBE3A expression in the paternally imprinted brain regions. The EEG of patients with Angelman syndrome reveals high amplitude spike-and-wave discharges, or rhythmic slowing which is maximal in the occipital region. Another well described neurogenetic disorder secondary to chromosome 15 pathology is Prader-Willi Syndrome. This condition is most often caused by a paternal interstitial deletion of a 6-Mb region of the chromosome 15q11-q13.

Rett syndrome is an X-linked dominant disorder caused by a mutation in the MeCP2 protein. In the United States, the prevalence of Rett syndrome is approximately 1 in 10,000 women. During the first 8 to 18 months of life, patients with Rett syndrome achieve developmental milestones as expected. Then, the children experience a plateau or even regression of development. Common features of patients with Rett syndrome include loss of communication skills, deceleration of head growth, loss-of-hand function, and stereotypic hand wringing. Other signs and symptoms of Rett syndrome include: breathing dysfunction (apnea and hyperventilation), bruxism, seizures, vasomotor instability, prolonged Q-T syndrome, and gait dyspraxia. Brain pathology in patients with Rett syndrome include mild to moderate cerebral atrophy, reduction or absence of pigmentation in the pars compacta of the substantia nigra, and decrease in the number of cells in the basal forebrain nuclei.

Velocardiofacial syndrome (VCFS) is caused by a micro-deletion at the q11.2 band on the long arm of chromosome 22. This anomaly results in defective development of the parathyroid glands, thymus, and conotruncal regions of the heart. A large number of these patients also have developmental delay, learning disabilities, and neuropsychiatric disorders (most notably schizophrenia). The conotruncal cardiac abnormalities in VCFS include: tetralogy of Fallot, truncus arteriosus, and interrupted aortic arch. VCFS is a specific syndrome that includes as part of its phenotype spectrum the DiGeorge sequence, the Pierre Robin sequence, and disorders associated with CHARGE syndrome.

Neurogenetic disorders that cause developmental delay include: (1) Miller Dieker syndrome (lissencephaly, chromosome 17p13); (2) subcortical band heterotopia (doublecortin gene, xq22.3); (3) polymicrogyria (1p36.3, PAXc6); (4) schizencephaly (10q26). The clinical presentation of these conditions is variable and includes dysmorphic features, mental retardation, epilepsy, learning disabilities, spasticity, and autism spectrum disorders.

Cerebral palsy (CP) is also a common cause of developmental delay. One of the earliest definitions of CP was coined by Mackeith and Polani in 1958. These authors indicated that CP is a condition of qualitative motor disorder appearing before the age of 3 years due to non-progressive damage to the encephalon. CP can also be defined as the consequence of a static or non-progressive lesion of the developing brain. Insults to the brain which cause CP occur in the pre- or perinatal periods. Children with CP may exhibit: motor impairment, cognitive impairment, speech-language delay, and impaired socialization ability. Based on the motor dysfunction, CP is classified as spastic, dyskinetic, atonic, or mixed. Rigidity and spasticity are the most common motor abnormalities seen in patient with CP. Medications used for the management of these signs include: baclofen, benzodiazepines, botulinum toxin injections, dantrolene, and tizanidine. Surgical management of rigidity and spasticity includes baclofen pump placement and selective dorsal rhizotomy.

In conclusion, the evaluation of a child for the chief complaint of developmental delay is labor intensive. As would be expected, the clinical suspicion guides the diagnostic work up. Tests that are commonly obtained include: MRI of the brain, CT scan of the head, comparative genomic hybridization, electroencephalogram, neuropsychological testing, and evaluation by occupational, physical, and speech-language therapist.

References

American College of Obstreticians and Gynecologists. Neonatal encephalopathy and cerebral palsy: defining the pathogenesis and pathophysiology. 2003. Washington DC.

Amir R, Van den Veyver I, Wan M, *et al.* Rett's syndrome is caused by mutations of X-linked methyl-CpG-binding protein. *Nature.* 1999.23:185–188.

de los Reyes EC, Roach ES. In: Andreoli T, Benjamin I, Griggs R, Wing E (eds.). *Cecil's Essential of Medicine.* Philadelphia: Saunder Elsevier. 2010. pp. 623–633.

Ferriero DM. Neonatal Brain Injury. *N Engl J Med.* 2004.35:1985–1995.

Lott I and Dierrsen M. Cognitive deficits and associated neurological complications in individuals with Down's syndrome. *Lancet.* 2010.9:623–633.

Manning M, Hudgins L. Array Based Technology and recommendations for utilization in medical genetics practice for detection of chromosomal abnormalities. *ACMG Practice guidelines.* 2010. Available at http://www.acmg.net/StaticContent/PPG/CMA_2010.pdf.

Shankaran S, Pappas A, Laptoook AR, *et al.* Outcomes of safety and effectiveness in a multicenter randomize clinical trial for whole body hypothermia for neonatal hypoxic ischemic encephalopathy. *Pediatrics.* 2008.122:e791–798.

Tan WH, Bacino Ca, Skiner SA, *et al.* Angelman syndrome: mutation influence features in early childhood. *Am J Med Genet A.* 2011. Jan.155A:81–90.

9

DUCHENE MUSCULAR DYSTROPHY

CY Tsao

A 3-year-old boy was evaluated by his pediatrician for the chief complaint of "frequent falls." The boy was born at term following an uncomplicated pregnancy. The child became able to roll from prone to supine and *vice versa* by 5 months of age. He, however, was not able to sit unaided until he was one year old. Similarly, he only became able to ambulate independently after age 2. Physical examination revealed the child to have prominent gastrocnemius muscles, and proximal muscle weakness in all extremities. When asked to stand up from the floor, the boy needs to roll over to face the floor, get on his knees, and use his hands to push on his thighs. The child's family history is significant for a maternal uncle who died of respiratory failure at the age of 18. The child's serum creatine kinase (CK) was 9,000 U/L (normal 0–235 U/L). Genetic evaluation revealed an out-of-frame deletion of exon 50 in the X-chromosome. The child's clinical history and laboratory profile are compatible with the diagnosis of Duchenne muscular dystrophy.

Introduction

Duchenne muscular dystrophy (DMD) is an X-linked recessive disease of muscle which is characterized by progressive loss of functional muscle mass and replacement with connective tissue. DMD is the most common form of X-linked muscular dystrophy. The incidence rate is estimated at 1/3500 live male births; *de-novo*

Division of Child Neurology, Nationwide Children's Hospital and The Ohio State University, Columbus, Ohio, USA

mutations are responsible for 30% of cases. Affected boys may come to medical attention for evaluation of clumsiness, wide-based gait and toe walking. Boys with DMD cannot run appropriately, have a lordotic gait, and when performing physical activities, are unable to keep up with their peers. The patients have difficulty walking up stairs and they need to use handrails for assistance. As the disease progresses, boys adopt a posture exhibiting increased lumbar lordosis and a wide based stance to increase stability. On physical examination, the patient's gastrocnemius muscles exhibit pseudohypertrophy. Also, when asked to stand up from sitting on the floor, patients utilize Gower's maneuver. In short, this sign is characterized by patients using their hands to "walk up the legs" so as to help lock the knees in place in order to bring the torso to the upright position. Once the diagnosis DMD is considered, it can be confirmed using laboratory tests. The serum level of creatine kinase (CK) in patients with DMD is greater than 10 times normal. Microscopic evaluation of the muscle biopsy of a boy with DMD will reveal significant muscle-fiber variability, signs of muscle necrosis and degeneration, and the presence of excessive amount of connective tissue. Immunostaining of the biopsy will fail to detect the presence of dystrophin. Finally, the diagnosis of DMD can be confirmed through DNA analysis. Such a test makes evident mutations within the dystrophin gene. Fifty to sixty-five percent of patients have deletions of one or more exons of the dystrophin gene; 5–10% patients have duplications of one or more exons; and 20–35% patients have small mutations. DMD is, at this time, a fatal disease. Most patients lose the ability to ambulate by age 12. Death occurs by the third decade of life secondary to cardiac and respiratory failure.

The differential diagnosis of DMD includes Becker muscular dystrophy, which is a milder form of DMD. The muscles of patients with Becker muscular dystrophy have the capacity to produce some dystrophin. As a consequence, patients with Becker muscular dystrophy usually continue to ambulate beyond 15 years of age. Other conditions to consider include the two types of limb-girdle muscular dystrophy (LGMD). LGMD type 1 is inherited in an autosomal dominant fashion; LGMD type 2 follows an autosomal recessive inheritance pattern. As the illness' name implies, patients with LGMD have weaknesses of the arms and legs. Serum CK level in patients with LGMD varies from normal to very high. Microscopic analysis of the muscle of patients with LGMD reveals normal distribution of dystrophin. However, sarcoglycans, calpain, dystroglycans, and other protein deficiencies have been associated with different types of LGMD.

At this time, there is no cure for DMD; treatments are aimed at delaying life threatening complications and improving patient's quality of life. The use of corticosteroids (prednisone, deflazacort) has been shown to provide transitory improvement of muscle strength. That in turn, translates into 1–2 more years of independent ambulation. The mechanism by which corticosteroids act in DMD is not well understood. Several theories to explain the effect, however, have been put forth: (1) corticosteroids suppress the inflammatory response and the resulting fibrosis, which occurs because of leakage of cell contents into the extracellular space; (2) corticosteroid stabilize the fragile myofiber membrane, thereby protecting the muscle from exercise-induced damage; (3) corticosteroids increase the regenerative capacity of the muscle allowing replacement of damaged muscle with new myofibers. Other potential treatment approaches for DMD include mutation suppression, exon skipping and gene replacement therapy.

Patients with DMD are at high risk for restrictive-obstructive thoracic disorder leading to hypoventilations and respiratory failure. The use of nasal bilevel positive airway pressure supports pulmonary function. Patients with DMD should be encouraged to receive the annual influenza vaccine. Prompt treatment of respiratory infections with antibiotics and chest physiotherapy are also indicated. The cardiac manifestations of DMD include arrhythmia and hypertrophic or dilated cardiomyopathy. Periodic evaluations by a cardiologist are highly recommended.

Resources for Patients

http://www.mda.org

References

Biggar WD, Gingras M, Fehlings DL, Harris VA, *et al.* Deflazacort treatment of Duchene muscular dystrophy. *J Pediatr.* 2001.138:45–50.

Bonifati MD, Ruzza G, Bonometto P, Berardinelli A, *et al.* A multicenter, double-blind, randomized trial of deflazacort versus prednisone in Duchene muscular dystrophy. *Muscle Nerve.* 2000.23:1344–1347.

Griggs RC, Moxley RT III, Mendell JR, Feichel GM, *et al.* Duchene dystrophy: randomized, controlled trial of prednisone (18 months) and azathioprine (12 months). *Neurology.* 1993.43:520–527.

Sussman M. Duchene Muscular dystrophy. *J Am Acad Orthop Surg.* 2002.10:138–151.

10

SPINAL MUSCULAR ATROPHY

CY Tsao

A 5-month-old boy is evaluated in the neurology clinic for the chief complaints of hypotonia and developmental delay. The child's mother indicates that, except for fewer fetal movements than she had expected, pregnancy, labor, and vaginal delivery were unremarkable. At 5 months of age, the child is yet to achieve head control. The child is also unable to roll over, and he cannot lift his arms or legs off the bed. On physical examination, the child is alert and makes good eye contact. He, however, has generalized muscle weakness in all extremities, hypotonia, and areflexia in addition to tongue fasciculations. There is no family history of neuromuscular or other neurological disorder. Genetic testing reveals homozygous deletion of exon 7 in the survival motor neuron 1 gene (SMN1). The clinical history, physical examination, and genetic testing are compatible with the diagnosis of type 1 SMA.

Introduction

Spinal muscular atrophy (SMA) is an illness characterized by progressive degeneration and loss of anterior horn cells (lower motor neuron) in the spinal cord and brainstem resulting in progressive muscle weakness. The incidence of SMA varies from 4-10/100,000 live births. Four types of SMA have been identified: prenatal, type I, type II, and type III. Progressive muscle weakness and normal cognitive abilities are the common denominators for all types of SMA. In prenatal type

Division of Child Neurology, Nationwide Children's Hospital and The Ohio State University, Columbus, Ohio, USA

SMA, weakness is recognized at birth; arthrogryposis multiplex congenita, and facial weakness may also be present. In type I SMA, patients present for evaluation around 3 months of age. Common findings on examination include: generalized muscle weakness, hypotonia, areflexia, and tongue fasciculations. These patients are unlikely to be able to sit unaided. Type II SMA usually becomes evident after age 6 months. As a general rule, these patients are eventually able to sit unaided; but they are unlikely to be able to walk without assistance. The physical examination reveals generalized weakness, hypotonia, and areflexia. Patients with type III SMA are usually diagnosed after 1 year of age. These patients are eventually able to walk unaided, but have proximal muscle weakness.

SMA is an autosomal recessive disorder. The gene mutation for all types of SMA is mapped to chromosome 5q11.2–13.3. The disease-causing gene is SMN1 (survival motor neuron 1), which codes for a full-length survival motor neuron protein necessary for normal function of the lower motor neuron. Homozygous deletions of exon 7 of SMN1 are seen in 95–98% of SMA patients. Approximately 2–5% of SMA patients are compound heterozygotes and have deletion of SMN1 exon 7 as well as a point mutation in SMN1.

Prior to the availability of genetic testing, the diagnosis of SMA was based on the clinical history plus the results of electrophysiological testing. The latter continues to be of use, especially when genetic testing is not available, it is deemed to be too costly, or the results are equivocal. Sensory and motor nerve conduction is, as a general rule, within normal limits. In contrast, electromyography is significantly abnormal. The test reveals signs of denervation and decreased motor action potentials. As expected, microscopic evaluation of muscle biopsies reveals atrophy of types 1 and 2 muscle fibers. Genetic evaluation of patients suspected of having SMA allows for rapid confirmation of the diagnosis and avoidance of unnecessary tests. The presence of three or more copies of SMN2 is associated with milder forms of SMA.

Prenatal SMA patients exhibit severe weakness and multiple joint contractures at birth; these patients usually die of respiratory failure before one month of age. Patients with SMA I have severe, generalized, progressive, and symmetric muscle weakness. They also have significant feeding difficulties. Without respiratory assistance such as bilevel positive airway pressure and gastrostomy tube feeding, patients with SMA I often die before age 2 years secondary to respiratory failure. With ventilatory support and adequate nutrition, patients with SMA I have survived into the 3rd decade of life. Patients with SMA II often lose the ability to sit independently during adolescence; up to 70% live beyond the 3rd decade of life. Patients with SMA III may lose the ability to walk independently during the 4th decade of life. That said they tend to have a normal life span.

The following disorders need to be differentiated from 5q SMA (SMN-associated SMA).

(1) Spinal muscular atrophy with respiratory distress 1. An autosomal recessive distal spinal muscular atrophy, linked to chromosome 11q13.2–q13.4 and associated with immunoglobulin mu-binding protein 2 gene mutation.
(2) Spinal muscular atrophy with pontocerebellar hypoplasia. An autosomal recessive disorder with spinal muscular atrophy and pontocerebellar hypoplasia.
(3) X-linked infantile spinal muscular atrophy. An X-linked spinal muscular atrophy with congenital contractures, hypotonia, and areflexia. Some patients have UBA1 gene mutations.
(4) Other disorders that require consideration include Pompe disease due to acid maltase deficiency, primary muscle disorders such as congenital myopathies, congenital muscular dystrophy, congenital myasthenic syndrome, and hexosaminidase A deficiency.

Treatment for SMA is mostly supportive. Poor weight gain and gastroesophageal reflux disease are common and require appropriate nutrition, gastric acid neutralizers, and promotility medications. In many cases, Nissen fundoplication and gastrostomy tube feeding become necessary. Secondary to ventilatory muscle weakness, the respiratory function of patients with SMA declines over time. Thus, patients benefit from chest physical therapy. In addition, bilevel positive airway pressure support helps avoid tracheostomy and relieves sleep disordered breathing. Some patients with SMA may require tracheostomy and mechanical ventilation. Scoliosis develops in patients with SMA types II and III; it may even be seen in those with SMA I who survive into the 2nd decade of life. Back braces do not prevent scoliosis, but can allow patients to sit upright. Surgical interventions are used to forestall further decline of respiratory function. Prophylactic immunizations for influenza, respiratory syncytial virus and streptococcus pneumoniae are extremely important for patients with SMA. Finally, the results of recent trials of medications such as valproic acid, hydroxyurea, and phenylbutyrate, used to improve activity of SMN2, seem to be promising. Stem cell therapy and gene therapy are also under active investigation as treatment for SMA.

Resources for Patients

www.mda.org (Muscular Dystrophy Association-USA)
www.projectcuresma.org (Project Cure SMA)
www.clinicaltrials.org (Clinical trial registry in USA)
www.enmc.org (European Neuromuscular Center)
www.pubmed.org (PubMed)

References

Han JJ, McDonald CM. Diagnosis and clinical management of spinal muscular atrophy. *Phys Med Rehabil Clin N Am.* 2008.19:661–680.

Lunn MR, Wang CH. Spinal muscular atrophy. *Lancet.* 2008.371:2120–2133.

Oskoui M, Kaufmann P. Spinal muscular atrophy. *Neurotherapeutics.* 2008.5:499–506.

Wang CH, Finkel RS, Bertini ES, *et al.* Concensus statement for standard of care in spinal muscular atrophy. *J Child Neurol.* 2007.22:1027–1049.

Wirth B, Brichta L, Hahnen E. Spinal muscular atrophy: from gene to therapy. *Semin Pediatr Neurol.* 2006.13:121–131.

11

MYASTHENIA GRAVIS

CY Tsao

A 3-year-old boy developed right eye ptosis 3 weeks after having a common cold. Two weeks later, the boy was reported to have difficulty going up a set of stairs. As a consequence, the boy was evaluated by a child neurologist and found to have bilateral ptosis, external ophthalmoplegia, and proximal muscle weakness in all extremities. The boy's parents reported that the ptosis and muscle weakness worsened in the afternoon and evening. While in the neurology ward, the boy received an IV injection of edrophonium. Within 15 seconds of the injection, the ptosis and ophthalmoplegia as well as the generalized muscle weakness resolved; the effect lasted 2 minutes. Additional testing revealed moderately elevated acetylcholine receptor antibody titers in the serum, and increased TSH and low T4 levels. Electrophysiological evaluation using 5-Hz repetitive nerve stimulation made evident a 15% decremental response of muscle action potentials. The boy was diagnosed as having myasthenia gravis (MG) and hypothyroidism. The boy was prescribed oral pyridostigmine every 4 hours and prednisone; within a few days, the above mentioned signs and symptoms resolved. The child was also placed on thyroid replacement therapy.

Introduction

MG is an acquired autoimmune disorder of the neuromuscular junction characterized by fluctuating muscle weakness and fatigability. The condition is induced by antibodies against the postsynaptic acetylcholine receptor of skeletal muscle. Some are induced by muscle-specific tyrosine kinase. In women, the condition usually

---

Division of Child Neurology, Nationwide Children's Hospital and The Ohio State University, Columbus, Ohio, USA

becomes evident during the 2nd or 3rd decades of life; and the 6th or 7th decades for men. The female to male ratio in both children and adults is 3:2. Prevalence of MG is 20–50/100,000; the annual incidence is 1–2/100,000. Transient neonatal MG occurs in 10–25% of babies born to mothers with MG. The symptoms usually last for a few weeks. The condition is a result of maternal antibodies crossing the placenta. Juvenile MG usually occurs in adolescents, but may also be seen in younger children.

According to the Clinical Classification of the American Myasthenia Gravis Foundation, there are five types of MG. Class I refers to instances where the patient has eye-muscle weakness exclusively. Class II indicates that the patient has eye-muscle weakness and *mild* weakness of other muscles; Class IIa indicates there predominantly is limb or axial muscle weakness; Class IIb indicates there predominantly is bulbar or respiratory muscle weakness. Class III refers to patients who have evidence of eye-muscle weakness and *moderate* weakness of other muscles; Class IIIa indicates there predominantly is limb or axial muscle weakness; Class IIIb indicates there predominantly is bulbar or respiratory muscle weakness. Class IV refers to those patients who have eye-muscle weakness and *severe* weakness of other muscles; Class IVa indicates predominant limb or axial muscle weakness; Class IVb indicates predominant bulbar or respiratory muscle weakness. Finally, Class V indicates the symptoms are so severe that the patient requires endotracheal intubation and mechanical ventilation.

In children with transient neonatal myasthenia gravis, the weakness may become evident during the first 3 days of life. Common findings are hypotonia, poor sucking and swallowing effort, and in severe cases, hypoventilation requiring mechanical respiratory support. The most common feature of juvenile myasthenia gravis is generalized muscle weakness which worsens with muscle activity and improves with rest. The initial symptoms may be swallowing difficulties, slurred speech, and ptosis, which can be uni- or bilateral. Ocular MG involves only the eye muscles. Generalized MG is that where muscle weakness is widespread. Ptosis, diplopia, unstable gait, facial weakness, dysphagia, and dysarthria may be present. Respiratory failure (myasthenic crisis) due to insufficient doses of medications requiring intubation may be seen during an infection, fever, stress, or adverse reaction to medications such as aminoglycosides, beta-blockers, lidocaine, procainamide, d-penicillamine and calcium channel blockers. A cholinergic crisis, due to excessive doses of medications, can induce flacid muscle paralysis, bronchospasm, profuse sweating, and cyanosis.

Serum acetylcholine receptor antibodies can be detected in 85% of patients with generalized MG, and 50% of those with ocular MG. Patients who do not have serum antibodies to acetylcholine receptors may, however, have antibodies against muscle specific kinase (MuSK). MuSK is a tyrosine kinase receptor which is required for the formation of the neuromuscular junction. Anti-striated muscle antibodies may also be detected in the serum, especially if a thymoma is present. Coexistence of MG with other autoimmune diseases such as Grave's disease and other autoimmune thyroiditis, rheumatoid arthritis, systemic lupus erythematosus, and polymyositis has been reported. Thus, it is important to measure the serum levels of thyroid hormones, thyroid stimulating hormone, anti-peroxidase antibody, rheumatoid factor, and antinuclear antibody in patients with MG. Patients with MG should also undergo a CT scan or magnetic resonance imaging of the chest to exclude the presence of thymus gland enlargement or thymoma. In patients with MG, the tensilon test induces rapid but temporary resolution of the symptoms. The benefit becomes evident within 30–45 seconds after an injection, and subsides within 3–5 minutes. Electrophysiological testing using 3-HZ repetitive nerve stimulation can induce $>10\%$ reduction in the amplitude of the compound motor action potential. Single fiber EMG has also been used to diagnose MG. In children presenting with ptosis, the differential diagnosis may include: botulism, stroke, cranial nerve palsy, mitochondrial disorder, multiple sclerosis, or congenital myopathy. In patients with acute onset of generalized weakness, it is important to rule out Guillain-Barre syndrome.

The signs and symptoms of transient neonatal MG may last a few weeks. They eventually subside once transplacental maternal antibodies have been removed from the child's bloodstream. Juvenile MG may remit within 2 years, but the signs and the symptoms of the condition wax-and-wane with infections, fever, stress, and some medications. In some instances, ocular MG subsides after a couple of years. In others, the condition progresses to become generalized MG.

A variety of medications are used to treat MG. The anticholinesterase pyridostigmine can be used at doses of 5 mg every 4 hours for patients with transient neonatal myasthenia. The dose is usually given 30 minutes before feeding via an NG tube until the symptoms subside. Alternatively, neostigmine 0.01–0.04 mg/kg intramuscular injection 30 minutes prior to feeding may also be used. For older children, pyridostigmine can be started at a dose 30 mg every 4–6 hours and be increased up to 7 mg/kg/day divided every 4–6 hours as tolerated. Prednisone at a dose of 1–2 mg/kg/day may improve muscle weakness in a few weeks; especially if pyridostigmine alone does not induce an appropriate response. The dose of prednisone can be gradually reduced over several months. Side effects from taking prednisone include: weight gain, hypertension, osteoporosis, irritability, cataracts, peptic ulcer, and a propensity to infections.

Intravenous immunoglobulin (IVIg), may directly neutralize the blocking effect of acetylcholine receptor antibodies. IVIg has been shown to provide significant benefit to patients with MG. A common protocol is to give patients 2 g/kg over 4 days every 4 weeks. Adverse effects of IVIg may include headache, fluid overload, aseptic meningitis, and renal failure. Plasmapheresis can remove pathogenic antibodies and cytokines and it is effective in severe generalized MG or pre-thymectomy in patients with respiratory of bulbar symptoms. A common protocol is to complete five plasma exchanges of 40–50 ml/kg over 9–10 days. Thymectomy is recommended for generalized myasthenia gravis and malignant thymoma, but not for patients with antibodies to MuSK because of lack of thymus pathology. Thymectomy has been done in children with severe generalized MG with good results.

Resources for patients:

www.myasthenia.org

References

Gold R, Schneider-Gold C. Current and future standards in treatment of myasthenia gravis. *Neurotherapeutics.* 2008.5:535–541.

Grob D, Brunner N, Namba T, *et al.* Lifetime course of myasthenia gravis. *Muscle Nerve.* 2008.37:141–149.

Herrmann DN, Carney PR, Wald JJ. Juvenile myasthenia gravis: treatment with immune globulin and thymectomy. *Pediatr Neurol.* 1998.18:63–66.

Selcen D, Dabrowski ER, Michon AM, Nigro MA. High dose intravenous immunoglobulin therapy in juvenile myasthenia gravis. *Pediatr Neurol.* 2000.22:40–43.

12

INHERITED NEUROPATHIES

Gloria Galloway

A 5-year-old girl is evaluated by the child neurologist for the chief complaints of weakness and deformity of her hands and feet. The child's parents indicate that 1 year before the evaluation, it had become evident that the child's legs were weak. She was unable to keep up with her peers, had difficulty going up a flight of stairs, and started developing high arched feet. As time went on, the child became unable to stand on her toes or on her heels. In addition to having high arched feet, she developed what was called "hammer toes." The child then began experiencing weakness of the hand muscles and a deformity that was described as "claw fingers." Upon examination, the child has weakness of the muscles of the foot and leg as well as the forearm and the hand. Deep tendon reflexes are absent in all extremities. The child's father indicates that he also has high arched feet and "hammer toes." The clinical history, family medical history, and results of electrophysiological testing are compatible with the diagnosis of hereditary motor sensory neuropathy also known as Charcot-Marie-Tooth disease.

Introduction

The inherited or hereditary neuropathies are a diverse group of conditions which are genetically and clinically diverse. The conditions, however, have as common denominators: peripheral nerve abnormities leading to weakness, pain, and deformity.

Division of Child Neurology, Nationwide Children's Hospital and The Ohio State University, Columbus, Ohio, USA

Based on clinical and genetic features, the inherited neuropathies can be classified into the following:

1. Hereditary motor sensory neuropathies (HMSN)
2. Hereditary sensory autonomic neuropathies (HSAN)
3. Giant axonal neuropathy
4. Multiple endocrine neoplasia
5. Infantile and juvenile neuroaxonal dystrophy
6. Familial amyloid polyneuropathy

Hereditary Motor Sensory Neuropathies (HMSN)

The most common inherited neuropathy is HMSN or Charcot-Marie-Tooth disease, with a prevalence of approximately 40/100,000. The condition encompasses a group of diseases with autosomal recessive, autosomal dominant, as well as X-linked inheritance. Patients with HMSN exhibit significant variation in the degree of clinical involvement and functional disability. Most often, the presenting complaint is distal weakness and foot deformity. Progressive weakness of more proximal muscles of the lower and upper extremities is characteristic, as is sensory loss. As the condition progresses, deep tendon reflexes become progressively more difficult to obtain; they usually disappear by the second decade of life. The feet of patients with HMSN have high arches, internal deviation, and hammer toes. Based on nerve conduction studies, HMSN can be classified into demyelinating, axonal, and pure motor forms.

Twenty-five gene mutations have been associated with HMSN; and the number continues to grow. Mutations in these genes can disrupt myelin formation, the neuron's cytoskeleton, axonal transport, the neuron's metabolism, and Schwann cell function. CMT1 is associated with a duplication on chromosome 17p11-2-p12. CMT1A is the most common form of CMT accounting for up to 50% of cases and is caused by the overexpression of PMP22, the peripheral myelin protein region on chromosome 17. CMT X1 is caused by mutations in the gap-junction B1 gene encoding for connexin-32; this form accounts for 10% of all cases of CMT. As with other conditions, the clinical features, suspected form of inheritance, and results of electrophysiological testing help guide the selection of genetic tests. CMT1A testing is indicated for patients who have evidence of demyelination on nerve conduction testing, and in whom the inheritance pattern appears to be either autosomal dominant or sporadic. Should these tests be unrevealing, and no male-to-male inheritance pattern be evident, testing for CMTX1 is reasonable. In instances where nerve conduction tests are compatible with the presence of an axonal form of CMT, testing for mutations in the MFN2 and MPZ genes is reasonable. If those tests are negative, CMTX1 evaluation can be considered. GDAP1 gene mutations are most commonly associated with autosomal recessive inheritance and should be done if suggested by the family history.

There is no specific treatment for CMT. Patients and their families benefit from genetic counseling, particularly for the purpose of family planning. Regular foot care helps prevent calluses and sores. The lifespan of patients with CMT is usually not affected, but there is significant variability in the amount of the disability present later in life. The authors of several studies have suggested the presence of "anticipation." That is, the condition becomes evident sooner in future generations. In such instances, symptom worsening leads to early functional disability. Co-morbid conditions significantly influence the severity of CMT and can affect functional disability and lifespan. For example, patients who develop diabetic neuropathy are much more affected than those who do not.

Hereditary Sensory and Autonomic Neuropathies (HSAN)

These are a group of inherited disorders of primary sensory and autonomic dysfunction. Associated features include plantar ulcers, syringomyelia, and altered threshold to pain and temperature. Several subsets of patients have been described depending on the suspected mode of inheritance and whether there is evidence of autonomic dysfunction.

HSAN 1 may be inherited in autosomal dominant, autosomal recessive, and X-linked forms. Patients with HSAN1 have sensory loss, foot ulcers, and mutilating acropathy. Onset is most often in adulthood. The lower extremities are more severely involved than the upper extremities. Patients with HSAN1 may exhibit plantar ulcers, pes cavus, sensory loss, symmetric leg weakness, muscle atrophy, restless leg syndrome, and lancinating limb pain. HSAN 2 is a condition that has either autosomal recessive or sporadic inheritance; symptom onset is during childhood. Patients with HSAN 2 may exhibit paronychia, ulcers of the fingers, sensory loss affecting all modalities, and diminished reflexes. Electrophysiological testing reveals absence of sensory nerve action potentials in distal portions of the limbs. HSAN 3 (dysautonomia) is an autosomal recessive form of HSAN which is more commonly seen in individuals with Jewish ancestry. The symptoms may be present at birth and they include: weak sucking reflex, swallowing difficulties, hypotension, profuse sweating, and respiratory distress. Later in life, many patients with HSAN 3 develop spine deformity. HSAN 4 is associated with insensitivity to pain, decreased ability to perceive other sensory modalities, anhydrosis, and cognitive impairment. HSAN 5 is associated with congenital loss of pain sensation.

Giant Axonal Neuropathy (GAN)

The clinical features of GAN include progressive clumsiness, distal muscle weakness and atrophy, areflexia, and sensory loss. Patients may also have kinky hair, foot deformities, cerebellar impairment, facial weakness, and scoliosis. Patients with GAN have mutations in the GAN gene (giant axonal neuropathy gene).

Multiple Endocrine Neoplasia Type 2B

This form of hereditary neuropathy is associated with medullary thyroid carcinoma, pheochromocytoma, ganglioneuromatosis, and abnormalities of skeletal and connective tissue.

Infantile and Juvenile Neuroaxonal Dystrophy

This is a severe neurodegenerative disorder in which death occurs during the first decade of life. Pathological features include the presence of axonal spheroids in the gray and white matter of the brain, and in the peripheral nerves.

Familial Amyloid Polyneuropathy

This is an autosomal dominant polyneuropathy associated with amyloid deposits in body organs and peripheral nerves. Familial amyloid polyneuropathy is a consequence of mutations in the transthyretin or TTR gene. Symptom onset is in early adulthood. Common manifestations include: cardiomyopathy, hypotension, urinary incontinence, and bowel dysfunction. Since transthyretin is produced in the liver, transplantation may be curative.

Treatment

Medical management of the inherited neuropathies involves several approaches. The first is aimed at preventing contractures and allowing the greatest range of motion at joints, stabilizing gait, and preventing falls. This aim is achieved with physical and occupational therapy involvement, use of orthotics if needed and tolerated, and use of assistive devices. Another aim is pain management. Pain in these cases is of neuropathic origin and described as burning, tingling or prickling sensations. Tolerance varies greatly among patients and in some no pharmacological intervention is needed. In others, the pain is not tolerable. In these cases pain management should avoid, if possible, narcotic use as this will be a long term intervention and narcotic use can lead to addiction and other adverse effects. Pharmacological interventions can involve the use of several anticonvulsant medications and antidepressant agents which have a neuropathic effect in pain control. The later can often be dosed once daily in the evening to lessen sedative effects. The former often requires titration to multiple doses in the day. The use of dietary supplements, particularly antioxidants, has been suggested. Randomized studies have not been done to support their use.

References

Amato A, Dumitru D. Hereditary neuropathies. In: *Electrodiagnostic Medicine.* 2nd ed. Philadelphia: Hanley and Belfus. 2002. pp. 889–936.

Carney JA, Chance P, Dyck PJ. Hereditary motor and sensory neuropathies. In: Dyck PJ, Thomas PK (eds.) *Peripheral Neuropathy.* 3rd ed. London: W B Saunders Company. 1993.

Daube J. *Clinical Neurophysiology.* 2nd ed. Oxford Press. 2002.

Dyck PJ, Lambert EH. Lower motor and primary sensory neuron diseases with peroneal muscular atrophy. II. Neurologic, genetic, and electrophysiologic findings in various neuronal degenerations. *Arch Neurol.* 1968.18:619–625.

Kacem A, Kefi M, Amouri R, Hentati F. Giant axonal neuropathy: clinical and genetic study in eight Tunisian families. *J Neuro Sci.* 2009.285;S143.

Kimura J. *Electrodiagnosis in Diseases of Nerve and Muscle: Principles and Practice.* 3rd ed. 2001. Oxford University Press.

Rosenburg R, Prusiner S, DiMauro S, Barchi R. *The Molecular and Genetic Basis of Neurological Disease.* 2nd ed. Boston: Butterworth-Heinemann. 1997.

13

ACQUIRED NEUROPATHIES

Gloria Galloway

Acquired Neuropathies

Acquired neuropathies are a group of conditions for which an identifiable cause is apparent. The symptoms become evident following exposure to the cause, although clinical progression may be slow as is the case in diabetes- and hypothyroidism-related neuropathies. Electrophysiological evaluation of a patient with an acquired neuropathy has evidence of focal or asymmetric abnormalities. Conduction block is one of the abnormalities that becomes evident through electrophysiological testing. Conduction block describes the inability of a nerve to fully conduct an action potential across an area, and it correlates to clinical weakness.

Electrophysiological testing may also make evident loss of response amplitude in the proximal segments of peripheral nerves. It may also make evident conduction velocity slowing and prolongation of distal latencies. In addition, there is reduction in the recruitment of motor units proximal to the site of injury. Clinical and electrophysiological features distinguish acquired neuropathies from those which are inherited. Based on etiology, acquired neuropathies can be classified as follows:

1. Neuropathies associated with altered immuno-modulation.
2. Neuropathies associated with infectious diseases.
3. Neuropathies associated with autoimmune connective tissue disorders.
4. Neuropathies associated with endocrine disease.
5. Neuropathies due to exposure to toxins.

Division of Child Neurology, Nationwide Children's Hospital and The Ohio State University, Columbus, Ohio, USA

6. Neuropathies associated with vitamin deficiencies.
7. Neuropathies associated with malignancies.

Neuropathies Associated with Altered Immuno-modulation

Guillain-Barre syndrome (GBS), also known as AIDP (acute inflammatory demyelinating polyneuropathy) was first described in 1859 by Landry as an acute ascending paralysis. The annual incidence of GBS is 1–4 per 100,000 with a peak age of onset between 30–40 years. In two-thirds of patients with GBS, symptom onset is preceded by a history of febrile illness. The most common infectious pathogen associated to GBS is *Campylobacter jejuni*. The signs and symptoms of GBS include paresthesia, dysesthesia, muscle weakness, decreased or absent deep tendon reflexes, and cranial nerve palsies. These abnormalities follow a distal to proximal progression. Of significant concern is respiratory failure as a consequence of diaphragmatic weakness. Laboratory evaluation of the cerebrospinal fluid of patients with GBS has evidence of elevated protein, with few or no white blood cells. In some patients, however, the protein level may be normal, particularly during the first week of the illness.

Electrophysiological evaluation of patients with GBS makes evident anomalies suggestive of demyelination with variable degrees of secondary axonal injury. Although the most common presentation of GBS is that of an ascending paralysis, a descending form may also occur; this is usually associated with ophthalmoparesis. Maximum weakness is reached within 2–4 weeks of symptom onset. Recovery follows a proximal to distal course and may happen over several months. The authors of multiple studies have shown improvement in the time course to recovery with the use of intravenous immunoglobulin and with plasmapheresis. Poor prognostic indicators include a distal compound action potential of $<10\%$ of normal; age >50 years; the need for assisted ventilatory support during the illness; and rapid onset of profound weakness. Peripheral neuropathy secondary to Lyme disease, HIV infection, sarcoidosis, cytomegalovirus, and Epstein-Barr virus may have similar presentation to GBS.

Variants of GBS

Acute motor-sensory axonal polyneuropathy

This is considered a variant of AIDP with predominant axonal involvement and poorer long term prognosis. Muscle weakness in patients with acute motor-sensory axonal polyneuropathy (AMSAN) progresses more rapidly, and the risk for respiratory compromise and autonomic disturbances including cardiac arrhythmias is higher than for patients with AIDP. Cerebrospinal fluid findings are similar to those of patients with AIDP but the electrodiagnostic studies usually reveal marked amplitude loss in both sensory and motor nerves likely due to conduction block.

Acute motor axonal polyneuropathy

This is another AIDP variant involving motor nerves with rapidly progressive symptom onset, respiratory compromise, and autonomic dysfunction. Cerebrospinal fluid findings are akin to those in AIDP and AMSAN. Electrodiagnostic studies make evident low amplitude or absent motor responses or CMAPS with sparing of sensory nerves.

Chronic inflammatory demyelinating polyneuropathy (CIDP)

This is a demyelinating polyneuropathy with a progressive or remitting and relapsing course. The condition's peak incidence is 40–60 years of age; 30% of patients have a history of an infectious process prior to symptom onset. Weakness is most often symmetrical. Treatment with IVIG or steroids can be used to improve the course of the neuropathy. A variant of CIDP is multifocal acquired demyelinating sensory and motor neuropathy or MADSAM. Patients with this condition experience asymmetric weakness with sensory loss and motor involvement of insidious onset. Some patients have elevated titers of ganglioside monosialic antibodies in serum (GMI); and like in other demyelinating neuropathies, protein level in the cerebrospinal fluid is elevated. The condition is treated with high dose steroids and IVIG infusions.

Distal-acquired demyelinating symmetric neuropathy (DADS)

Patients with this polyneuropathy have little or no distal weakness. They do, however, exhibit distal sensory loss and reduced or absent deep tendon reflexes. Electrodiagnostic studies reveal signs of demyelination. The serum of patients with DADS has high titers of anti-myelin–associated glycoproteins (anti-GAD). The response of patients with DADS to immunomodulating treatment is modest.

Multifocal motor neuropathy

This demyelinating polyneuropathy involves motor nerves with sensory nerve sparing and may or may not be associated with conduction block. Often, there is focal muscle weakness that typically begins in the upper extremities; muscle cramps and fasciculations are common. Weakness is asymmetric and muscle atrophy may be present. Although the condition is immune mediated, the protein levels in the cerebrospinal fluid is typically normal. Over 80% of patients with multifocal motor neuropathy have elevated titers of IgM antibodies, particularly anti-GMI antibodies. IVIG can be used for treatment in these patients with some success. Rituximab adjunctive treatment along with IVIG may offer some reduction in disability scores and improved muscle strength outcome.

Vasculitic neuropathy

This is an acquired polyneuropathy in which there is perivascular inflammation and blood vessel necrosis. Patients also have signs of peripheral nerve involvement including mononeuropathy multiplex, distal symmetric polyneuropathy and bilateral mononeuropathy multiplex. Pathological evaluation of peripheral nerves makes evident loss of nerve fibers within and between nerve fascicles. Electrodiagnostic studies make evident a decrease in action potential amplitude of both sensory and motor nerves with relatively normal nerve conduction velocity. For non-systemic vasculitic neuropathy treatment, recommendations from the Peripheral Nerve Society Guideline include the use of corticosteroids for 6 months as monotherapy followed by combination therapy with immunosuppressive agents including cyclophosphamide, azathioprine, or methotrexate as IV pulses. Once in remission, maintenance therapy with azathioprine or methotrexate for 18–24 months may be used.

Neuropathies Associated with Infectious Diseases

Treatment is directed at resolution of the underlying infectious disorder when possible.

Leprosy neuropathy

Leprosy neuropathy, caused by *Mycobacterium leprae*, is found worldwide. The condition has three clinical forms:

(1) Tuberculoid leprosy in which a cell-mediated immune response causes well-defined, circumscribed granulomatous lesions that involve the skin and superficial nerves. This form of leprosy causes clinical features similar to those of a mononeuropathy multiplex.
(2) Lepromatous leproasy is characterized by impairment of cell-mediated immunity, resulting in widespread and intense infection. The clinical features include skin rash, skin discoloration, and loss of eyebrows and eyelashes. This form, of leprosy is characterized by a symmetric and progressive sensory polyneuropathy.

(3) In borderline forms of leprosy, there is impaired cell-mediated immunity. Patients with this form of leprosy exhibit sensorimotor polyneuropathy or mononeuropathy.

Electrophysiological manifestations of all forms of leprosy neuropathy include: decreased or absent sensory nerve action potentials, and slow conduction of motor action potential. The electromyogram reveals the presence of abnormal spontaneous muscle discharges.

HIV and HTLV1

HIV and HTLV1 infections may be associated with mononeuropathies, but these are less common in pediatric patients. That said, the symptoms may be present early in life due to *in utero* exposure. Various forms of HIV- and HTLV1-related neuropathy have been described, including forms resembling AIDP, CIDP, mononeuropathy multiplex, and polyneuropathy with autonomic features.

Lyme infection

The condition, caused by the spirochete *Borrelia burgdorferi*, may be associated with various forms of neuropathy including distal peripheral neuropathy, ADIP-like polyneuropathy, mononeuropathy multiplex, and polyradiculoneuropathy. Cranial neuropathies especially facial nerve palsy, may also occur. Electrophysiological studies make evident a decrease in amplitude of both sensory and motor nerve action potentials. Microscopic examination of a nerve biopsy reveals the characteristic perivascular infiltration of plasma cells and lymphocytes.

Neuropathies Associated with Autoimmune Connective Tissue Disorders

These neuropathies can be associated with Sjogren syndrome, rheumatoid arthritis, systemic lupus erythematosus, scleroderma, and mixed connective tissue disease. Common electrodiagnostic features of these conditions include distal sensory > motor axonal neuropathy or axonopathy. In Sjogren syndrome, the patient characteristically presents with sicca complex: dry eyes, dry mouth, and occasionally dryness of other mucus membranes. Sjogren syndrome-related neuropathy is present in 10–15% of patients and may be the presenting complaint. Rheumatoid arthritis-related neuropathy usually presents late in the disease's progression. Electrodiagnostic studies reveal a mild sensory neuropathy. Sarcoidosis is a granulomatous disorder affecting multiple organs including the liver, spleen, parotid glands, mucous membranes, and the central and peripheral nervous systems. Patients present with fever, cough, weight loss, and fatigue. Cranial nerve involvement may occur in a mononeuropathy multiplex pattern; facial nerve paresis is common. The most common electrodiagnostic features of the disorder is loss of amplitude of sensory responses in a mononeuropathy multiplex pattern. Treatment for the abovementioned disorders can be challenging as the agents used for neuropathic pain alleviation are often not effective, and yet, they may cause iatrogenic complications.

Neuropathies Associated with Endocrine Diseases

Diabetic neuropathy

This condition is most commonly characterized by a slowly progressive distal symmetric sensory and motor polyneuropathy. Other forms include: an asymmetric polyradiculoneuropathy, focal and multifocal mononeuropathies of the limbs and cranial nerves, and an autonomic neuropathy which is often associated with variable degrees of sensory neuropathy. Clinical features include lancinating pain, and a burning sensation along with impairment of other sensory modalities involving the feet and distal portions of the leg. Absence of deep tendon reflexes is common, particularly in patients with a demyelinating form of the condition. Electrophysiological tests make evident varying degrees of demyelination and axonal damage. Changes which become evident early in the disease process include: reduction in the amplitude of the sensory nerve action potential, conduction velocity slowing, and prolongation of the latency. Sympathetic skin testing and quantitative sudomotor axon reflex testing (QSART) are helpful diagnostic tools which may reveal abnormalities before changes in routine nerve conduction test becomes evident.

Hypothyroidism neuropathy

This condition usually presents as a mononeuropathy. The most common manifestation of the condition is carpal tunnel syndrome, and the second most common is tarsal tunnel syndrome. Hypothyroid neuropathy may also be associated with demyelinating predominantly distal polyneuropathy similar to diabetic polyneuropathy.

Uremic neuropathy

This condition may be associated with a sensorimotor polyneuropathy or multiple mononeuropathies, often in the setting of renal failure.

Other systemic disorders that may have an associated polyneuropathy include: neuropathy secondary to liver disease, critical illness polyneuropathy, and neuropathy associated with gout, chronic obstructive pulmonary disease (COPD), and gastrointestinal disorders. Treatment in these disorders is directed at improvement of the underlying endocrine disorder.

Neuropathies Secondary to Toxin Exposure

Included in this group are: (1) neuropathy secondary to chemotherapeutic agent exposure, most notably vincristine, cisplatin, and taxol; and (2) neuropathy secondary to antimicrobial agents including metronidazole and chloroquine. In many instances, the neuropathy is a consequence of a dose-dependent response. Also in this category of neuropathies are those due to exposure to toxic agents such as solvents and industrial chemicals. Electrophysiological evaluations of patients with neuropathy secondary to toxin exposure reveal a sensorimotor polyneuropathy predominantly axonal and distal.

Neuropathies Associated with Vitamin Deficiencies

Deficiencies of vitamins B12, B6, B1, and E may be associated with a sensory-motor neuropathy characterized by burning dysesthesia, ataxia, distal weakness, and atrophy. Decrease in the amplitude of the sensory nerve action potential is characteristic of these neuropathies. The electromyogram may have evidence of muscle fiber irritability.

Neuropathies Associated with Malignancies

These neuropathies may either be a consequence of the direct effect of the malignancy on the peripheral nervous system or they may be secondary to remote effects of the neoplasm (paraneoplastic neuropathies). Lymphomas can cause neurological abnormalities including cranial nerve palsies, spinal cord damage, and peripheral neuropathies. The results of electrophysiological evaluations correlate with the clinical features; both sensory and motor nerves may be involved. Paraneoplastic neuropathies are most commonly associated to carcinomas of the lung. They have, however, also been described in association with carcinoma of the gastrointestinal tract, the breast, and the prostate. Most commonly, a sensory motor neuropathy is seen; but pure sensory neuropathies have been described. Symptoms include dysesthesia and distal muscle weakness. As paraneoplastic neuropathies mimic those caused by other conditions, search for an underlying malignancy is indicated. It is not uncommon for the neuropathy to be diagnosed prior to discovery of the underlying malignancy.

References

Amason B, Loiven B. Acute inflammatory demyelinating polyradiculoneuropathy. In: Dyck J, Thomas PK (eds.) *Peripheral Neuropathy.* 3rd ed. London: W B Saunders Company. 1993.

Amato A, Dumitru D. Acquired neuropathies. In: Dumitru D, Amato A, Zwarts M (eds.) *Electrodiagnostic Medicine.* 2nd ed. Texas: Hanley & Belfus. 2001. pp. 937–1042.

Birbaum J. Peripheral nervous system manifestations of Sjogren syndrome: clinical patterns, diagnostic paradigms, etiopathogenesis, and therapeutic strategies. *Neurologist.* 2010.16:287–297.

Collins M, Dyck J, Gronseth G, *et al.* PNS NSVN Guideline on the classification, diagnosis, investigation, and immmunosuppresive therapy of non-systemic vasculitic neuropathy: executive summary. *J Peripher Nerv Syst.* 2010.15:176–184.

Daube J. *Clinical Neurophysiology.* 2nd ed. Oxford Press. 2002.

Kimura J. *Electrodiagnosis in Diseases of Nerve and Muscle: Principles and Practice.* 3rd ed. Oxford University Press. 2001.

Reik L. Peripheral neuropathy in Lyme disease. In: Dyck J, Thomas PK, (eds.) *Peripheral Neuropathy.* 3rd ed. London: W B Saunders Company. 1993.

Sabin T, Swift T. Jacobson R. Leprosy. In: Dyck J, Thomas PK (eds.) *Peripheral Neuropathy.* 3rd ed. London: W B Saunders Company. 1993.

Thomas PK, Tomlinson DR. Diabetic and hypoglycemic neuropathy. In: Dyck J, Thomas PK (eds.) *Peripheral Neuropathy.* 3rd ed. London: W B Saunders Company. 1993.

14
PEDIATRIC STROKE

Warren Lo

Introduction

Stroke in children was once considered a rare disorder, but increasing clinical attention and the wider availability of imaging technologies have led to a growing recognition that childhood stroke is more common than originally thought. The general term "stroke" encompasses ischemic brain injury due to thrombotic or embolic occlusion of cerebral arteries or veins, and hemorrhagic brain injury from subarachnoid or intraparenchymal hemorrhage. If an ischemic neurological deficit disappears within 24 hours, that deficit is termed a transient ischemic attack (TIA), although a proportion of patients with TIAs of that duration will have evidence of cerebral infarction on neuroimaging studies. In the following sections, I review the clinical manifestations, causes, diagnostic evaluation, and treatments of pediatric ischemic and hemorrhagic stroke.

Recent epidemiological studies reflect the wider use of magnetic resonance brain imaging (MRI), which has made the detection of ischemic stroke and arterial vasculopathy much easier. The authors of a population-based study that combined medical records and radiology information reported an incidence of 2.4 ischemic strokes/100,000 children after the neonatal period. The investigators used an identical approach and found an incidence of non-traumatic hemorrhagic stroke to be 1.7 cases/100,000 patients. Together, these data yield a collective incidence of ischemic and hemorrhagic stroke of 4.1/100,000. The proportion of hemorrhagic to ischemic stroke in these two studies (41%) was similar to what we found from

Division of Child Neurology, Nationwide Children's Hospital and The Ohio State University, Columbus, Ohio, USA

an administrative dataset that was statistically adjusted to cover the entire US. In that study, we found that hemorrhagic stroke accounted for 45% of all strokes in children ages 30 days to 20 years. Taken together, these studies suggest that hemorrhagic stroke accounts for 40–45% of childhood stroke.

The frequency of stroke in the newborn is higher than in older children and the incidence of ischemic stroke in term neonates approaches that of older adults. Analysis of the US National Hospital Discharge Survey from 1980 through 1998 revealed that the incidence of neonatal ischemic stroke is 17.8/100,000 and an incidence of hemorrhagic stroke is 6.7/100,000. A population-based estimate of hemorrhagic stroke in term infants found an annual incidence of 6.3/100,000, similar to that previously reported.

Clinical Manifestations

Neonatal AIS

Ischemic stroke in neonates can be difficult to detect, which is why a proportion of children have a delayed diagnosis of presumed perinatal stroke. If newborns present with focal seizures, and they come to evaluation promptly, subtle alterations of consciousness or subtle motor deficits alone may be missed or dismissed as non-specific. The full clinical picture of focal seizures, focal motor deficits, and an altered level of consciousness should suggest an ischemic or hemorrhagic stroke. Other conditions that should be considered include: focal trauma, subdural hemorrhage, meningitis, herpes encephalitis, and inborn errors of metabolism.

Childhood AIS

Arterial ischemic stroke results from occlusion of one or more arteries by thrombosis or embolism. The classic presentation of a thrombotic stroke is a stuttering, gradual deficit that progresses over minutes to hours. An embolic stroke is sudden and more fulminant, with the deficit rapidly reaching its peak. If an embolus breaks up, the deficit may suddenly improve, although this is uncommon. The location of the occlusion determines the clinical manifestations.

Anterior circulation infarctions

Occlusions of the internal carotid artery and the middle cerebral artery result in similar findings unless collateral flow across the anterior communicating attenuates the effect of an internal carotid occlusion. Both arterial syndromes present with contralateral hemiparesis and hemisensory loss. Internal carotid artery occlusion tends to cause a dense impairment of face, arm, and leg, and a dense contralateral visual field cut. If the left hemisphere is affected, there will be a dense aphasia while involvement of the right hemisphere results in neglect. Middle cerebral artery occlusion causes a milder deficit, with relative sparing of the leg. The visual field may not be affected, and aphasia or neglect may be milder. Internal carotid and extensive middle cerebral artery ischemia can result in extensive brain edema and increased intracranial pressure. Patients with large strokes are at substantial risk for brain herniation.

Anterior cerebral artery occlusion is uncommon, but when it occurs, there typically is weakness in the contralateral leg, cognitive impairment, incontinence, and apraxia. In a normal anatomic variant, both anterior cerebral arteries arise from a common trunk so that infarction can cause bilateral leg weakness with little involvement of the face and arms. In that case, infarction of both frontal lobes may result in bowel and bladder incontinence, decreased spontaneity, distractibility, and emotional lability. The recurring artery of Heubner originates from the anterior cerebral artery. Occlusion will cause infarction of the head of the caudate and the anterior corpus callosum, resulting in facial and hand weakness, dysarthria, transcortical aphasia, and verbal memory dysfunction.

Lenticulostriate (lateral striate and medial striate) arteries are small terminal branches of the middle cerebral artery that supply the lateral and medial aspects of the lentiform nucleus (putamen and globus pallidus), caudate, and the anterior limb of the internal capsule. Infarction results in a severe motor hemiparesis with or without dysarthria and variable sensory involvement.

Posterior circulation infarctions

The thalamogeniculate branches of the posterior cerebral artery and the posterior communicating artery supply the lateral and posterior thalamus. Infarction in the region supplied by the posterior communicating artery may result in a pure hemisensory stroke that may include a homonymous quadrantanopsia, and memory disturbance. Infarction in the region supplied by the posterior cerebral artery may result in the thalamic syndrome of contralateral loss of pain and temperature perception, and positive motor phenomena including tremor, myoclonus, chorea, akathisia, and ataxia. The medial portion of the thalamus is supplied by midbrain paramedian arteries. Occlusion of these vessels results in impaired consciousness, hemiparesis, hemiataxia, vertical gaze palsy, memory loss, confusion, and hemi-neglect.

The posterior cerebral arteries, are branches of the basilar artery. They supply the occipital lobes and variable portions of the posterior temporal and parietal lobes. Infarction usually causes a contralateral homonymous hemianopia that may spare a portion of the macular vision since that may be supplied by the middle cerebral artery. Infarction of the posterior aspects of the corpus callosum and occipital lobe results in contralateral hemianopia plus the inability to read but with preserved writing ability.

Occlusion of flow from the basilar artery to the posterior cerebral arteries will infarct the midbrain and a variable extent of one or both occipital lobes resulting in hemianopia or cortical blindness accompanied by ocular motility disorders. Infarction of the midbrain, red nucleus, and the superior cerebellar peduncle may result in a cranial nerve III palsy, contralateral ataxia and involuntary movements, and contralateral weakness. Infarction of the ventral midbrain usually involves cranial nerve III with pupillary dilation and lack of light responsiveness, oculomotor paresis, and contralateral weakness involving the lower half of the face. Dorsal midbrain infarction results in paralysis of up gaze, convergence-retraction nystagmus, eyelid retraction, and large pupils with light-near dissociation.

A lesion of the superior lateral pons results in ipsilateral ataxia, contralateral hemiplegia and contralateral sensory loss depending upon the level of the infarct. In the lower pons, a lateral lesion results in ipsilateral loss of facial sensation. Bilateral infarction of the ventral pons results in the locked-in syndrome, notable because the patient is quadriplegic and unable to speak. The patient is fully conscious and can see, hear, and feel. Vertical eye movements are intact. Infarction of the lower ventral pons results in contralateral hemiplegia not affecting the face. Occlusion of the antero-inferior cerebellar artery results in infarction of the lateral lower pons and the undersurface of the cerebellum. This is manifested by ipsilateral ataxia, ipsilateral facial nerve weakness, and there may be an inability to look conjugately towards the side of the lesion.

Occlusion of the posterior inferior cerebellar artery results in infarction of the lateral medulla, inferior cerebellar peduncle, and inferior cerebellum. This is manifested by hoarseness, dysphagia, diminished gag, and ipsilateral palatal paralysis. The patient may have an ipsilateral Horner syndrome, nausea, nystagmus, vertigo, dysarthria, and ipsilateral ataxia. Hiccups, contralateral loss of pain and temperature sensation, and mild weakness are variable. Infarction of the medial medulla may result in contralateral hemiplegia sparing the face, contralateral loss of proprioception and vibratory perception, and ipsilateral tongue paralysis.

Transient ischemic attacks (TIAs)

Transient ischemic deficits are uncommon in children. Yet, they are likely underdiagnosed. The clinical deficits are similar to the ischemic strokes described above, but the findings are transient and often clear within minutes to hours. In children, TIAs may result from small emboli or local hemodynamic factors which temporarily impair adequate perfusion. Magnetic resonance brain imaging may help identify old small infarctions or areas of acute diffusional abnormalities even in patients whose clinical dysfunction resolved completely within a few hours. Such patients need treatment to reduce the risk of recurring infarcts even though they do not have clinical signs or symptoms.

Cerebral sinovenous thrombosis (CSVT)

Thrombosis of a cortical vein, dural sinus, or deep cerebral vein may be silent or symptomatic although the findings may be less apparent than with an arterial occlusion (Figure 1). If the thrombosis produces increased intracranial pressure, patients may present with the features of pseudotumor cerebri — increased intracranial pressure, headache, papilledema, and cranial nerve deficits. If venous occlusion produces cerebral infarction, the patient may present with focal neurological findings or seizures.

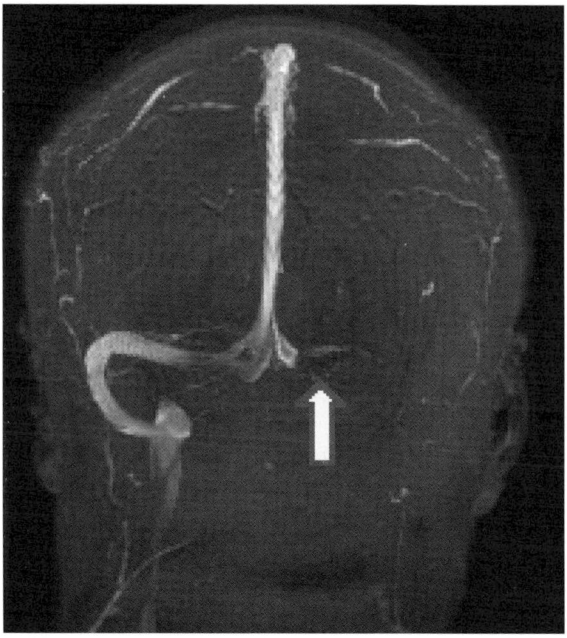

Figure 1. Magnetic resonance venogram. Three-dimensional reconstruction demonstrates a sinovenous thrombosis with occlusion of the left transverse sinus marked by the arrow.

Presumed perinatal ischemic stroke (PPIS)

Children with delayed recognition of a PPIS typically present in early infancy (2–4 months) when the parents recognize that the child is not using one arm or one side of the body as much as the other. Even then, if the finding is subtle and the parents or healthcare providers wait to see if the deficit spontaneously clears, then evaluation may be delayed. The onset of focal seizures or infantile spasms typically leads to a more timely evaluation. Some children have such subtle deficits that they may not be diagnosed until a radiological study is ordered for a different purpose.

Hemorrhage

The typical presentation of an intracerebral hemorrhage is the sudden onset of headache, altered mental status, nausea and vomiting, focal neurological signs, and occasionally seizures (Figure 2). Very young children cannot report headache and nausea, so they may present with non-specific signs such as mental status changes and seizures. These two signs may occur in a third of the children with brain hemorrhage. Overall, the clinical picture depends upon the hemorrhage's size and location; small hemorrhages in the frontal lobe may have surprisingly few signs.

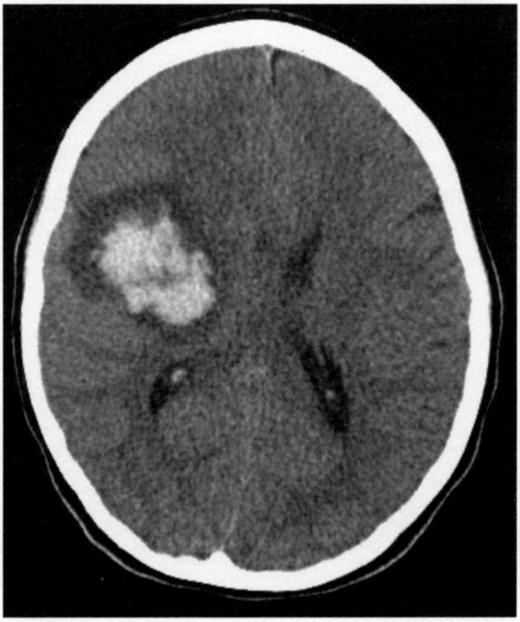

Figure 2. CT scan showing a intracerebral hemorrhage with a surrounding rim of edema.

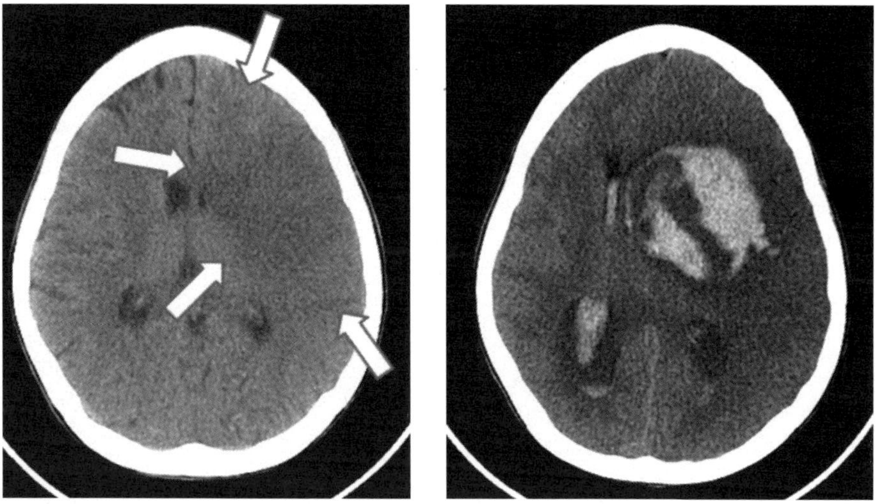

(a) (b)

Figure 3. (a) CT scan shows an acute ischemic infarct of the left frontal lobe. Note the loss of the gray-white junction and sulcal markings delineated by the arrows. (b) CT scan 48 hours later shows hemorrhagic conversion of the ischemic infarct and blood in the ventricles.

Severe subarachnoid hemorrhage presents with sudden, severe headache, vomiting, meningismus, and a variable alteration of consciousness. Subarachnoid hemorrhage with small amounts of blood may be limited to irritability rather than an obvious alteration of consciousness. Emesis and photophobia can be present with relatively little meningismus. Retinal hemorrhages support the clinical diagnosis, but these may be difficult to detect in an uncooperative child.

These hemorrhages noted here are different from the hemorrhagic conversion of an ischemic infarct (Figure 3). A mild degree of hemorrhagic conversion will not alter the initial neurological findings from the ischemic stroke. A moderate to large hemorrhagic conversion can result in increased brain edema and new neurological signs. A venous infarction that has few clinical signs may become apparent when a hemorrhagic conversion induces seizures.

Etiology of Stroke

One major reason to search for an etiology is to identify a potential cause of stroke recurrence. Some causes of ischemic and hemorrhagic stroke are listed in Tables 1 and 2.

Table 1. Risk factors for ischemic stroke in children.

- **Cardiac disease**
  - *Congenital*
    - Valvular
    - Complex heart disease
  - *Acquired*
    - Endocarditis
    - Cardiomyopathy
- **Hematologic disorders**
    - Sickle cell disease
- **Pro-thrombotic states**
  - *Genetic thrombophilias*
    - Antithrombin III deficiency
    - Factor V Leiden mutation
    - Hyperhomocysteinemia
    - Protein S deficiency
    - Protein C deficiency
    - Prothrombin mutation
  - *Acquired*
    - Thrombotic thrombocytopenic purpura
    - Thrombocytosis
    - Polycythemia
    - Oral contraceptives
    - Pregnancy/postpartum period
    - Disseminated intravascular coagulation (DIC)
    - l-Asparaginase
    - Systemic malignancies
    - Leukemia
    - Nephrotic syndrome
    - Hemolytic-uremic syndrome
    - Autoimmune diseases
      - Lupus anticoagulant
      - Anticardiolipin antibodies
      - Inflammatory bowel disease
- **Vasculopathies**
  - Focal cerebral arteriopathy
    - Transient
    - Progressive
  - Varicella
  - Dissection
  - Moyamoya
  - Fibromuscular dysplasia

(*Continued*)

Table 1. (*Continued*)

Vasculitis
Primary CNS vasculitis
CNS vasculitis with autoimmune disease
Systemic lupus erythematosus
Polyarteritis nodosa
Takayasu's arteritis
Rheumatoid arthritis
Dermatomyositis
Infections
Meningitis
Encephalitis (herpes simplex)
Mastoiditis
Otitis
Tonsillitis
Intravenous drug abuse
Metabolic
Mitochondrial encephalopathies
MELAS
PDHC deficiency
Homocystinuria
Fabry disease
Drugs
l-Asparaginase
Steroids
Trauma
Traumatic embolus (fat, air)
Traumatic dissection
Surgery
Cardiac
Head, neck, carotid artery
ECMO
Cardiac or cerebral catheterization
Migraine

Causes of ischemic infarction

Advances in neuroimaging technology allow for non-invasive inspection of craniocervical vessels. In turn, there is growing realization that arterial lesions (vasculopathy) are important causes of stroke and may account for up to one-third of ischemic strokes. Focal vasculopathy can occur as a consequence of varicella

Table 2. Risk factors for intracranial hemorrhage in children.

Intracranial vascular anomalies
Arteriovenous malformation
Cavernous malformation
Aneurysm
Brain tumor (primary or metastatic)
Coagulopathy
Clotting factor deficiencies
Congenital
Hemophilia (factor VIII or factor IX deficiency)
Factor VII (proconvertin) deficiency
Factor XIII (fibrin-stabilizing factor) deficiency
Afibrinogenemia
Acquired
Disseminated intravascular coagulation
Liver failure
Warfarin therapy
Vitamin K deficiency
Anticoagulant/thrombolytic/antiplatelet agents
Thrombocytopenia
Genetic
Acquired
Systemic malignancies and chemotherapeutic agents
Miscellaneous
Hemorrhagic conversion of an ischemic infarction
Herpes simplex encephalitis
Drug related (amphetamines, cocaine, PCP, others)

infection, may be an initial manifestation of moyamoya syndrome, or may be idiopathic. Dissection of the carotid or vertebral arteries may be spontaneous, traumatic, or may occur in patients with fibromuscular dysplasia or collagen disorders such as Ehlers-Danlos type IV. Since dissection may occur outside of the cerebral circulation, if there is clinical suspicion of a dissection, for example multiple infarcts of varying ages, imaging studies should specifically examine the extracranial, i.e. cervical carotid or vertebral arteries (Figure 4).

Congenital or acquired heart disease can be identified in up to 30% of children with a stroke. Complex congenital heart disease accounts for the largest proportion of these patients. The role of a patent foramen ovale as a cause for stroke in children and young adults is controversial. Clinical studies are currently being performed

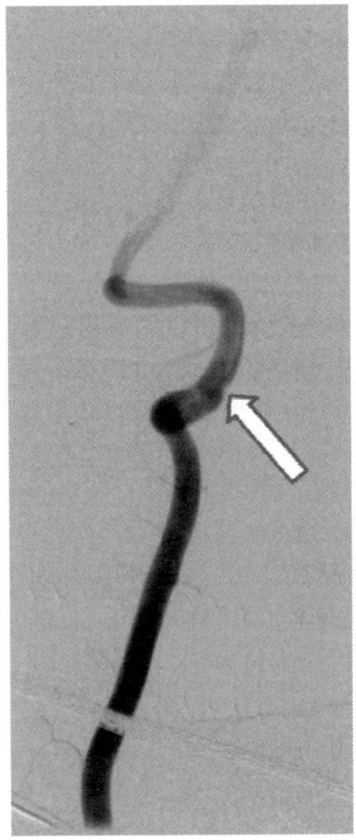

Figure 4. Catheter angiogram demonstrating a subtle dissection of the vertebral artery (white arrow) in a patient with multiple cerebellar and posterior temporal infarcts.

to address this question, but the available data suggest that closure does not affect the recurrence of ischemic stroke in young adults with a PFO.

Before routine ultrasound screening of cerebral blood flow, about a fourth of individuals with sickle cell disease developed symptomatic ischemic infarctions and at least half developed silent infarcts. Monitoring and chronic transfusion programs have reduced this frequency. Children between 2 and 5 years of age have the highest risk of ischemic stroke, but stroke can occur at any age. Another complication of sickle cell disease is a moyamoya-like vasculopathy which can cause ischemic stroke in children and hemorrhagic stroke in adults.

The role of thrombophilias in the genesis of stroke is complex. Certain gene mutations are common in the general population, such as factor V Leiden or methylene tetrahydrofolate reductase, and the detection of a heterozygous mutation does not immediately translate into a higher risk for recurring thromboembolism. A number of the thrombophilias, such as antithrombin III deficiency or prothrombin mutation are associated with an increased risk of venous thromboembolism, but their link to arterial thrombosis is less robust. Certain proteins such as antithrombin III, protein C and protein S are consumed during acute thrombosis so an abnormally low level needs to be followed up when the patient is stable. With these cautions in place, patients with new onset ischemic or hemorrhagic stroke should be evaluated for a clotting disorder. If abnormalities are found, they need to be discussed with hematologists who deal with clotting disorders.

Causes of sinovenous thrombosis

Thrombosis of a cortical vein or dural sinus often occurs in an individual with a hypercoagulable state (Table 1). The likelihood of a venous thrombosis is greater in individuals with adjacent infections such as meningitis, encephalitis, chronic otitis, sinusitis or orbital cellulitis. Other risk factors include thrombophilias, hemoglobinopathy, polycythemia, and dehydration. It goes without saying that individuals may have multiple risk factors.

Causes of hemorrhage

Intracranial vascular anomalies such as arteriovenous malformations, cerebral aneurysms, and cavernous malformations are collectively the most common risk factor for non-traumatic brain hemorrhage in children (Table 2). If one aggregates the results of several case series, over half occurred in children with an intracranial vascular anomaly and these children have a high risk of recurrence. Other children may have thrombocytopenia or coagulation defects. Hemorrhage into a brain tumor is a common cause of hemorrhagic stroke.

Diagnostic Evaluation

Risk factor evaluation

While the cause of a stroke may sometimes appear obvious, such as the case with sickle cell disease or congenital heart disease, a careful search for other risk factors is warranted. The initial evaluation should include simple non-invasive tests with low cost and high yield. A complete blood count may identify polycythemia, hemoglobinopathy, infections, or thrombocytopenia. Hemoglobin electrophoresis should be done on patients at risk for sickle cell disease who have not been already tested. A sedimentation rate, prothrombin time, and partial thromboplastin time and fibrinogen should be included. For new-onset ischemic stroke, one should assay antithrobmin III, protein S, protein C, factor V Leiden, prothrombin mutation, serum homocysteine, thrombin time, and anticardiolipin IgM and IgG. Patients who have had hemorrhage should have fibrinogen and d-dimer levels measured in addition to the prothrombin time and the partial thromboplastin time.

Congenital and acquired cardiac lesions are important causes of ischemic stroke. An electrocardiogram and echocardiogram should be obtained as well as a consultation from a pediatric cardiologist. In a child with a slim habitus, a trans-thoracic echocardiogram usually yields sufficient information to exclude an embolic source. A stouter child may need a transesophageal study. The significance of a patent foramen ovale is still being investigated, but data in young adults have not shown that closure of a PFO reduces the risk of recurrence.

In the setting of fever, a child with an acute focal neurological deficit should undergo a lumbar puncture if there is no evidence of significant mass effect. Herpes simplex encephalitis can present with a subacute infarct and the diagnosis may be evident only by PCR analysis of the cerebrospinal fluid. Tuberculous meningitis, syphilitic meningitis, or HIV encephalitis can present with stroke. Autoimmune vasculitis may be difficult to diagnose, but a CSF pleocytosis without fever may provide a clue, particularly in the presence of multifocal infarcts.

Radiographic evaluation

The presence of an ischemic stroke can usually be confirmed early in the illness with the diffusion sequence (and perfusion sequence when available) of a magnetic resonance brain scan (MRI). The presence of intracranial hemorrhage can be detected with MRI or CT scan. The MRI may be less available than CT, and the acquisition of all MRI sequences may require patient sedation.

MR angiography (MRA) provides a non-invasive means to image intracranial vessels (Figure 5). The MRA is extremely useful for patients in whom the diagnosis of a vasculopathy is suspected but not definite. The limitations of MRA are: the test is less sensitive than catheter angiography to small arterial disease, the test may overestimate a focal constriction, and the test can miss subtle dissections. The detection rate based on CT angiography (CTA) for large and medium vessels approaches that of catheter angiography, and this modality is becoming more widely available. The high amount of radiation (currently the exposure of one CTA equals that of 10 regular CT scans) raises concerns regarding the long-term effects of ionizing radiation. Some recommend that CTA not be performed in young children.

The sensitivity question is less critical for venous obstruction, so that MR venography (MRV) and CT venography (CTV) are equally applicable and can be differentiated on availability, need for sedation, and radiation exposure. Both modalities are sufficient to detect obstruction in the large sinuses and

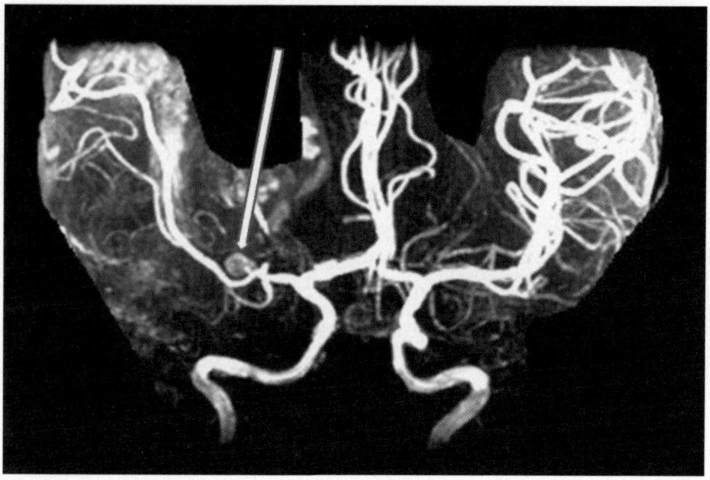

Figure 5. Magnetic resonance arteriogram. Three-dimensional reconstruction demonstrates a mycotic aneurysm (thin white arrow) in a child with subacute bacterial endocarditis.

deep internal cerebral veins. Occlusion of small veins can be missed by both techniques, but the susceptibility-weighted sequence that is now becoming available for MRI helps identify regions of venous stasis at the level of the internal cerebral veins.

Catheter angiography remains the "gold standard" for evaluation of smaller intracranial arteries and detecting subtle changes in larger vessels. If there is a high level of suspicion that a vascular lesion may have caused the patient's ischemic or hemorrhagic stroke, a normal MRA or CTA should not preclude a catheter angiogram.

Treatment of Stroke in Children

The treatment of pediatric stroke involves acute and chronic measures. The goal of acute treatment is to minimize the extension of any initial damage, treat an underlying disease, and prevent acute recurrence. In the chronic phase, the goal is to prevent stroke recurrence, promote motor and coordination recovery, and promote recovery of cognitive and behavioral function. Several excellent reviews address treatment in detail. Recent treatment guidelines were developed by the consensus of expert panels. They are limited by the lack of data from randomized clinical trials (RCTs). The one exception is that data from RCTs show chronic transfusion therapy reduces stroke recurrence in children who have sickle cell disease and who are at risk for ischemic stroke.

Acute management: General measures

Preserving brain homeostasis is essential to minimize further damage. This is accomplished by assuring an adequate supply of oxygen and nutrients, and minimizing unnecessary metabolic demands.

Supportive measures are similar for acute ischemic stroke, sinovenous thrombosis, and intracranial hemorrhage. A patient who had an acute stroke is at risk for brain edema, herniation, aspiration, and hypoventilation. Supportive care must include airway protection and adequate oxygenation, and monitoring the level of consciousness by staff with experience in neurological diseases. Aspiration may be difficult to detect, so one should maintain a high level of suspicion and if in doubt, test the adequacy of swallowing and oro-pharyngeal reflexes. Fluid homeostasis requires careful monitoring of vital signs, intake and output, and perfusion. One should avoid fluid restriction that results in poor cardiac output and decreased cerebral perfusion, but one also should avoid fluid overload that will exacerbate cerebral edema.

Clinical deterioration, particularly a deteriorating level of consciousness, warrants transfer to an intensive care unit that can provide intracranial pressure monitoring (ICP), and if possible, measurement of cerebral blood flow and cerebral blood oxygenation. There is no data to show hypothermia improves outcome from stroke, but fever increases cerebral metabolism, therefore fever should be controlled so that the patient is normothermic. Blood pressure should be managed judiciously, with the primary concern to maintain cerebral perfusion pressure. An elevated blood pressure may be a homeostatic response to preserve cerebral perfusion pressure via cerebral autoregulation; so that overly aggressive treatment of mild to moderate hypertension may induce cerebral hypoperfusion. Severe elevation of blood pressure may promote rebleeding from an aneurysm; judicious lowering of the blood pressure is appropriate. There is no evidence that lowering of the blood pressure will reduce clot expansion with an intracerebral hemorrhage (ICH).

Convulsive and non-convulsive seizures can increase cerebral metabolic rate and cerebral oxygen consumption. Patients with ischemic stroke who have not manifested seizures usually do not need routine prophylaxis with anti-seizure medication. Neonates are an exception as seizures may be the presenting sign of a stroke; and neonates may have multiple seizures, status epilepticus, and non-convulsive seizures. Convulsive seizures can increase the risk of rebleeding from an aneurysm or arteriovenous malformation (AVM), so prophylaxis with anti-seizure medication even without symptomatic seizures is reasonable. Since the level of consciousness may be a key clinical sign, one may consider using less sedating anti-seizure medications such as phenytoin, levetiracetam, or valproic acid (where age appropriate) rather than phenobarbital. If a patient is paralyzed to assist with mechanical ventilation or if there is a persistent, and unexpected impairment of consciousness, one should consider the possibility of non-convulsive status epilepticus.

If there is no clinical evidence for increased ICP and a supratentorial infarct is small, the patient can be managed conservatively. A large hemispheric infarction or a large intracerebral hemorrhage can produce sufficient brain edema to severely compress adjacent brain tissue. A lesion in the posterior fossa can result in severe brainstem compression or obstruction of cerebrospinal fluid drainage and secondary obstructive hydrocephalus. Patients with these types of strokes need close monitoring for signs of increasing ICP or brain herniation and should be managed aggressively. A decreasing level of consciousness or other signs of neurological deterioration such as an evolving asymmetric pupil should lead to a quick assessment for brain herniation, and ICP monitoring.

There are multiple means to treat increased ICP, all of which have limitations. Intubation and hyperventilation to a pCO_2 of 30–35 mm Hg can reduce ICP, but the effect is temporary and hyperventilation to a pCO_2 below 30 mm Hg can decrease cerebral blood flow. Treatment with intravenous mannitol (0.5–1.0 gm/kg/dose) and hypertonic saline can reduce ICP, but these measures last only hours to a few days. Ventriculostomy and cerebrospinal fluid drainage should be performed if there is acute hydrocephalus. Surgical evacuation of a posterior fossa hemorrhage, or resection of infarcted cerebellar tissue may be life-saving. The authors of small case series in children have demonstrated that emergency hemicraniectomy may be a life-saving measure in the event of a large hemispheric or MCA distribution infarct.

Acute management: To prevent stroke recurrence

The etiology of ischemic stroke in children is usually different from that in adults since atherosclerosis is unlikely. Instead, cardiac embolism, vasculopathy, or sickle cell disease are more likely causes. The goal of acute treatment is to reduce the risk of early stroke recurrence. The authors of consensus guidelines recommend initial anticoagulation with unfractionated heparin (UFH) (Schedule I) or low molecular weight heparin (LMWH) (Schedule II) for children suspected of having a high risk of recurrent cardiogenic embolism, patients with a severe hypercoagulable state, and individuals with an acute vasculopathy. Relative contraindications to anticoagulation include intracranial bleeding and a large infarct with a high risk of hemorrhagic conversion. Anticoagulation is not recommended for an intracranial dissection because these individuals may develop a subarachnoid hemorrhage. The need for acute anticoagulation can be reconsidered after an evaluation for a specific cause. If no cause has been found or if the recurrence is low, for example an embolic stroke after catheterization or cardiac surgery, then acute anticoagulation may be shifted to an anti-platelet agent. If a potential risk factor such as a vasculopathy, uncorrectable congenital heart lesion, or severe thrombophilia have been identified, treatment can be shifted to warfarin (Schedule III; target INR of 2.0–3.0) or low-molecular weight heparin for 3–6 months.

If anticoagulation is not suitable, aspirin may be started at a dose of 3–5 mg/kg/day, and adjusted downward to 1–3 mg/kg/day if the higher dose is not tolerated (Schedule IV). Aspirin is often prescribed in children in an effort to prevent recurrent stroke following TIA. Other antiplatelet agents, dipyridamole and clopidogrel, are used, but safety and efficacy data in children are nonexistent.

Acute management: Once a source for potential recurrence is identified

Vasculopathies

Arterial dissection: For extracranial dissection the patient should be anticoagulated acutely with UFH or LMWH and then converted to (a) warfarin with a target INR of 2.0–3.0; (b) LMWH; or (c) an antiplatelet agent for chronic treatment lasting 3–6 months depending upon the healing of the vessel. If the dissection involves an intracranial vessel, there is an increased risk for subarachnoid hemorrhage. In that case, one must weigh the benefit of anticoagulation to prevent further embolization versus the risk of hemorrhage.

Focal arteriopathies: The recurrence risk for ischemic stroke remains significant for years. Treatment similar to that for arterial dissection seems reasonable, with initial use of low-molecular weight heparin and transitioning to antiplatelet agents for extended time. Monitoring of the vasculopathy is important since some large vessel stenoses may worsen or progress to moyamoya syndrome.

Congenital heart disease: For an acute non-infections embolus considered to have a high risk of recurrence, anticoagulate with UFH or LMWH then convert to warfarin or continue LMWH for an extended time or until the lesion heals. For an acute non-infectious embolus considered to have a low or unknown risk of recurrence, treat with aspirin for perhaps one year. Because of the risk of hemorrhage following a septic embolus, patients with infectious endocarditis should not be anticoagulated.

Prothrombotic disorders: If a risk factor is associated with recurring stroke such as severe persistent protein C or antithrombin III deficiency, then anticoagulate with UFH or LMWH with plans to convert to warfarin or LMWH for 3–6 months.

The role of some risk factors regarding recurrence may be unclear and will need reassessment when the patient is stable. A heterozygous genetic mutation may not be the same as a significant thrombophilia. Hematology consultation may be appropriate.

Sickle cell disease: Acutely provide adequate hydration and oxygenation. Acutely transfuse if the total hemoglobin is below 10 g/dl, then exchange transfuse the patient to reduce the HbS below 30% of the total Hgb. The patient should then progress to chronic transfusion for chronic management. The presence of sickle cell vasculopathy may require medical therapy before proceeding to a surgical option.

Cerebral sinovenous thrombosis: In the case of an occlusion with acute neurological symptoms, assure appropriate hydration, treat seizures if present, and treat elevated ICP if present. Anticoagulate with UFH or LMWH followed by chronic LMWH or transition to warfarin. Mild intraparenchymal hemorrhage does not contraindicate anticoagulation and there is evidence that anticoagulation reduces the risk of thrombus propagation. A large hemorrhagic infarct should be managed cautiously. In selected individuals, directed thrombolysis may be considered. Others, especially those without symptoms may be observed with follow-up imaging of the venous system; extension of the thrombus may compel one to anticoagulate.

Intracranial hemorrhage: Intracranial hemorrhage due to warfarin therapy may be treated with intravenous vitamin K, fresh frozen plasma, prothrombin complex concentrate, or recombinant factor VIIa depending upon the size and location of the bleeding. Patients receiving heparin can be treated with protamine sulfate. Unfractionated heparin can be fully reversed with protamine sulfate; low-molecular weight heparin is reversed only 70%. It is important to remember that measures to stop further hemorrhage pose risks of thromboembolic complications. Large cerebellar hemorrhage (>3 cm in adults) which causes brainstem compression or hydrocephalus should be evacuated early. A small cerebellar hemorrhage where there is no brainstem compression can be managed medically. Given the frequency of intracranial vascular lesions as a cause of hemorrhage and the risk of re-bleeding with these lesions, surgical or intravascular techniques to correct the lesions should be considered. Occlusion of an aneurysm should be pursued early to reduce the risk of early re-bleeding. Calcium-channel blocking agents, such as nimodipine, may benefit vasospasm due to subarachnoid hemorrhage (SAH) although the evidence for their efficacy is weak and there is no data regarding efficacy in children.

Additional measures for acute arterial ischemic stroke

There is little information about the effectiveness or risks of thrombolytic agents in children. There are multiple published case reports of children who have been treated with tissue plasminogen activator (tPA). There are, however, no data regarding safety and efficacy, nor dosing guidelines in children.

Chronic treatment to prevent stroke recurrence in specific conditions

Arterial dissection: Continue chronic treatment with (a) warfarin with a target INR of 2.0–3.0; (b) LMWH; or (c) antiplatelet agent for 3–6 months until the vessel wall has healed as determined by follow-up imaging studies. If the vessel wall does not heal by 6 months, one may consider tapering medication off and observing; the rate of recurrence in adults has been reported to be low. In children, there are no clear guidelines or how long treatment should last. If despite anticoagulation and antiplatelet therapy stroke or TIA(s) recur, an interventional or surgical approach may become necessary.

Vasculopathy without dissection: These patients need regular neuroimage monitoring of the vasculopathy, since some evolve to more severe unilateral involvement or moyamoya syndrome. The approach is similar to that of arterial dissection: antiplatelet agents, anticoagulation and then surgery if there is stroke recurrence, TIA, or progressive vasculopathy on medical therapy.

Moyamoya syndrome: Revascularization procedures such as direct or indirect bypass have been advocated to prevent progression of symptoms. The key is to perform revascularization before a severe stroke occurs. Revascularization surgery should be considered when there are progressive signs and symptoms of ischemia, or when cerebral blood flow or cerebral perfusion reserve are inadequate. If a patient is being managed without revascularization surgery, aspirin prophylaxis should be used. If one follows a patient conservatively, one needs to monitor for the occurrence of ischemic symptoms such as a TIA. The vessel appearance will need to be followed regularly, but one should remember that MRA can overestimate a stenosis. Cerebral blood flow can be monitored by non-invasive techniques such as SPECT, PET, or perfusion MRI. If moyamoya syndrome is detected as an incidental finding, there is little evidence to guide the timing of a bypass procedure. The limited available outcome data in children suggests that functional outcomes are poor in those who are not treated surgically, but that provides no guidance regarding timing.

Congenital heart disease: To reduce stroke recurrence, heart failure should be treated, atrial myxoma should be resected, and cardiac defects should be repaired. Major atrial septal defects should be closed. Until then, long-term anticoagulation should be considered if the risk of repeat embolization is high; anti-platelet agents may be considered if the risk is low. After a defect has been surgically repaired, it is reasonable to continue aspirin for 6 months. The role of a patent foramen ovale as a mediator of stroke in the young is controversial. Limited evidence in adults suggests that closure does not reduce an already low rate of recurrence.

Prothrombotic disorders: After 3–6 months of chronic warfarin or LMWH, the duration of treatment should be reviewed. The appropriate duration of anticoagulation is unknown, and some acute deficiencies of protein C and S or antithrombin III may be transient therefore in specific patients, observation off treatment after initial anticoagulation may be reasonable.

Sickle cell disease: Children aged 2 to 16 years who have a confirmed cerebral infarction should have periodic RBC transfusions to suppress the HgbS level. Surgical revascularization procedures may be considered in children with SCD who have a moyamoya-like vasculopathy and persistent cerebrovascular dysfunction despite optimal medical management.

Cerebral sinovenous thrombosis: Anticoagulation with LMWH or warfarin for 3–6 months is reasonable as determined by the speed of vascular recanalization or the recurrence of a thrombosis. If the thrombosis is present after 6 months of therapy, discontinuation of anticoagulation should be considered.

Chronic management of hemorrhagic stroke

If a source of bleeding can be identified, it should be treated to reduce the risk of recurrence. The authors of a population-based study examined risk factors for recurring hemorrhagic strokes in children. Most recurrences occurred within the first 6 months after the incident hemorrhage. There were no recurrences in children who had idiopathic hemorrhagic stroke. Children who had structural lesions such as AVMs or CNS tumors had a recurrence rate of 13% and children who had underlying medical causes had a recurrence rate of 13%. The latter group had recurrence within a week of the initial hemorrhage.

Endovascular management of aneurysms and arteriovenous malformations have been used since the early 1990s. There is less information regarding has newer endovascular techniques such as stents and angioplasty in the management of ischemic strokes in children; although sporadic case reports indicate that these procedures are performed in children. In subarachnoid hemorrhage due to an aneurysm, prompt intervention with coils should be considered to reduce the risk of early rebleeding. The disadvantage with coils is that in adults only 50–70% of aneurysms are completely occluded, and up to 33% of coiled aneurysms will regrow.

Trends in rehabilitation

The authors of the recent randomized control trial of constraint-induced movement therapy (CIMT) in adults (EXCITE) showed that intensive training and physical therapy of the affected arm while constraining the unaffected arm resulted in sustained improved upper-limb function in moderately affected patients. The authors showed that, 2 weeks of intensive physical therapy resulted in better function than standard treatment, and this improved function was present for up to 1 year after treatment. The authors of recent reviews have suggested that CIMT has not been tested rigorously in children. The field of pediatric cerebrovascular disease is evolving quickly, but current data consist of small trials, case series, or case reports. The authors of a recent Cochrane review of CIMT in children with hemiplegic cerebral palsy pointed out the limitations of the published studies and suggested that CIMT in children with hemiplegic cerebral palsy should be considered experimental rather than truly therapeutic.

Schedule for the Dosing of Unfractionated Heparin (UFH)

UFH often requires dosage adjustments that may take several days to achieve target prolongation of the APTT; however, UFH can be rapidly reversed with protamine sulfate or fresh frozen plasma.

- Start 20 units/kg/hr; (Some clinicians use a loading dose of 75 U/kg IV over 10 mins; others use no bolus/loading dose)
  - Infants: 28 U/kg/hr
  - Children (>1 year of age): 20 U/kg/hr
  - Older children: 18 U/kg/hr (similar to adults)
- Titrate to APTT 60–80 sec
- Monitor APTT 4 hrs after every dose change until therapeutic, then daily (with CBC to check platelets)
  - Adjustments
  - APPT sec < 50 Increase rate by 10% (Some will give a bolus 50 U/kg)
  - APPT sec 50–59 Increase rate by 10%
  - APPT sec 60–85 No change
  - APPT sec 86–95 Decrease rate by 10%

— APPT sec 96–120 Hold infusion 30 mins, decrease rate by 10%
— APPT sec >120 Hold infusion 60 mins, decrease rate by 15%

Schedule for the Dosing of One Form of Low-Molecular Weight Heparin (LMWH)

LMWH can quickly achieve suitable levels of anticoagulation and require fewer lab tests. However, LMWH cannot be reversed as completely as UFH. Other LMWHs exist (eviparin, dalteparin, and tinzaparin).

- Enoxaparin subcutaneous injection dosing
  - Infants < 2 months:
    - Initial treatment: 1.5 mg/kg/dose twice daily
    - Initial prophylaxis: 0.75 mg/kg/dose twice daily
  - Infants > 2 months – children 18 years:
    - Initial treatment: 1 mg/kg/dose twice daily
    - Initial prophylaxis: 0.5 mg/kg/dose twice daily
  - Anti-factor Xa assay target level is 0.5–1.0 u/mL [Treatment]
    - Draw blood 4 hours post injection
    - Reduce dose in severe renal failure

Schedule for Warfarin Dosing

- Day 1 if INR is 1.0–1.3, 0.2 mg/kg/day orally
- Loading Day 2-4
  - INR 1.1–1.3 Repeat initial loading dose
  - INR 1.4–1.9 50% of initial loading dose
  - INR 2.0–3.0 50% of initial loading dose
  - INR 3.1–3.5 25% of initial loading dose
  - INR > 3.5 Hold dose until INR is < 3.5 then restart at 50% of the previous dose
- Maintenance
  - INR 1.1–1.4 Increase by 20% of dose
  - INR 1.5–1.9 Increase by 10% of dose
  - INR 2.0–3.0 No change
  - INR 3.1–3.5 Decrease by 10% of dose
  - INR > 3.5 Hold dosing until INR is < 3.5 then restart at 20% less than previous dose

Schedule for Antiplatelet Agent Dosing

Aspirin dosing ranges from 1–5 mg/kg/day. Starting dose 3–5 mg/kg/day. If the patient does not tolerate the high dose then try decreasing to 1–3 mg/kg/day.

Adult studies suggest that aspirin doses ranging from 30–150 mg/day are sufficient to reduce the risk of ischemic stroke, and there is no benefit to doses greater than 300 mg/day. If stroke recurs on aspirin monotherapy, the combination of aspirin 75 mg and dipyridamole is more effective for secondary stroke prevention.

Clopidogrel is an alternative for those with aspirin hypersensitivity. Adult dosing is 75 mg/day.

References

Agrawal N, *et al.* Imaging data reveal a higher pediatric stroke incidence than prior US estimates. *Stroke.* 2009.40:3415–3421.

Albers GW, *et al.* Antithrombotic and thrombolytic therapy for ischemic stroke: *American College of Chest Physicians Evidence-Based Clinical Practice Guidelines.* 8th Edition. *Chest.* 2008.133(6 Suppl):630S–669S.

Estan J, Hope P. Unilateral neonatal cerebral infarction in full term infants. *Arch Dis Child Fetal Neonatal Ed.* 1997.76:F88–F93.

Fullerton HJ, *et al.* Recurrent hemorrhagic stroke in children: a population-based cohort study. *Stroke.* 2007.38:2658–2662.

Ganesan V, *et al.* Investigation of risk factors in children with arterial ischemic stroke. *Ann Neurol.* 2003.53:167–173.

Govaert P, *et al.* Perinatal cortical infarctation wihtin middle cerebral artery trunks. *Arch Dis Child Fetal Neonatal ED.* 2000.82:F59–F63.

Halkes PH, *et al.* Aspirin plus dipyridamole versus aspirin alone after cerebral ischaemia of arterial origin (ESPRIT): randomised controlled trial. *Lancet.* 2006.367: 1665–1673.

Hennekens CH, *et al.* Dose of aspirin in the treatment and prevention of cardiovascular disease: current and future directions. *J Cardiovasc Pharmacol Ther.* 2006.11: 170–176.

Monagle P, *et al.* Antithrombotic therapy in neonates and children: American College of Chest Physicians Evidence-Based Clinical Practice Guidelines (8th Edition). *Chest.* 2008.133(6 Suppl):887S–968S.

Monagle P, *et al.* Antithrombotic therapy in children: the seventh ACCP conference on antithrombotic and thrombolytic therapy. *Chest.* 2004.126(3 Suppl):645S–687S.

Pediatric Stroke Working Group. Stroke in childhood: clinical guidelines for diagnosis, management, and rehabilitation. 2004. Royal College of Physicians. www.rcplondon.ac.uk/pubs/books/childstroke.

Perkins E, *et al.* The cost of pediatric stroke acute care in the United States. *Stroke.* 2009.40:2820–2827.

Roach ES, *et al.* Management of stroke in infants and children: a scientific statement from a Special Writing Group of the American Heart Association Stroke Council and the Council on Cardiovascular Disease in the Young. *Stroke.* 2008.39:2644–2691.
Switzer JA, *et al.* Pathophysiology and treatment of stroke in sickle-cell disease: present and future. *Lancet Neurol.* 2006.5:501–512.

15

NEUROCUTANEOUS SYNDROMES

Monica Islam and E. Steve Roach

A 4-month-old infant is brought to the neurology clinic for evaluation. For the past week, the child has exhibited quick contractions of his arms and legs that occur in clusters. The child has had normal development to date. The physical examination is notable for a heart murmur and a hypopigmented patch on his right shin.

A 5-year-old child is brought to the neurology clinic. The parents have noted the child to be squinting and bumping into objects. Examination of the skin reveals multiple hyperpigmented macules and freckles in her axillae. These skin findings have been present since infancy but have increased in number and are more visible in the summer.

Introduction

Each of these patients has tell-tale neurological signs and symptoms that raise concern for a neurocutaneous syndrome: tuberous sclerosis in the first case and neurofibromatosis type 1 in the second. Neurocutaneous syndromes are congenital or hereditary conditions that feature lesions of both the skin and nervous system. Although each condition is distinct and characterized by a unique pathophysiology, the concept of neurocutaneous syndromes unifies those

Division of Child Neurology, Nationwide Children's Hospital and The Ohio State University, Columbus, Ohio, USA

time of diagnosis, these patients should have an MRI of the brain to assess tuber burden and screen for subependymal giant cell astrocytomas (SEGAs) that can lead to obstructive hydrocephalus. Evaluation of the kidneys with ultrasound or MRI is critical to monitor for renal angiomyolipomas and other renal tumors. Unlike SEGAs and renal tumors that are likely to increase in number and size with time, cardiac rhabdomyomas are likely to involute with age. A screening echocardiogram at the time of diagnosis should suffice unless there are other symptoms or abnormalities. Ophthalmologic examinations are needed to monitor for retinal hamartomas. Regarding pulmonary involvement, all symptomatic patients and asymptomatic females by age 18 years require evaluation with CT of the chest. Molecular genetic testing in the form of sequence analysis or deletion/duplication analysis is helpful in diagnosing individuals with atypical features and in identifying a disease-causing mutation that can be passed to other children.

Neurofibromatosis 1

Affecting approximately 1 in 3000 individuals, neurofibromatosis type 1 (NF-1) is the most common neurocutaneous syndrome. Its most serious complications affect the nervous system. The cutaneous manifestations are often prominent, with *café-au-lait* macules (Figure 2a), axillary freckling, and superficial neurofibromas that often increase in size and number with age. The inheritance of NF-1 is autosomal dominant, but approximately half of those affected result from *de novo* mutations. The gene on the long arm of chromosome 17 is large, and numerous mutations have been documented. The *NF1* gene product, neurofibromin, is a tumor-suppression GTPase-activating protein that inhibits *ras*-mediated cell proliferation. Not all individuals with NF-1 have obvious neurofibromas, while others have hundreds. Most of these are small and therefore asymptomatic, but larger lesions can create symptoms related to neuropathy as well as structural susceptibility to injury (such as friction of a neurofibroma against clothes). Plexiform neurofibromas are more likely to cause symptoms and disfigurement. In the lumbosacral region, for example, they can grow large enough to cause obstructive hydronephrosis. These otherwise benign tumors have potential for transformation into malignant peripheral nerve sheath tumors. Other manifestations of NF-1 include Lisch nodules and pseudoarthrosis. Pseudoarthrosis of a dysplastic long skeletal bone can raise concern for the diagnosis of NF-1 at birth. Identification of a second diagnostic criterion (such as an affected first-degree family member) is necessary to confirm the diagnosis. *Café-au-lait* spots typically arise in infancy, and it is important to remember that a few *café-au-lait* spots can be present in unaffected individuals. Most children with six or more *café-au-lait* spots might eventually meet

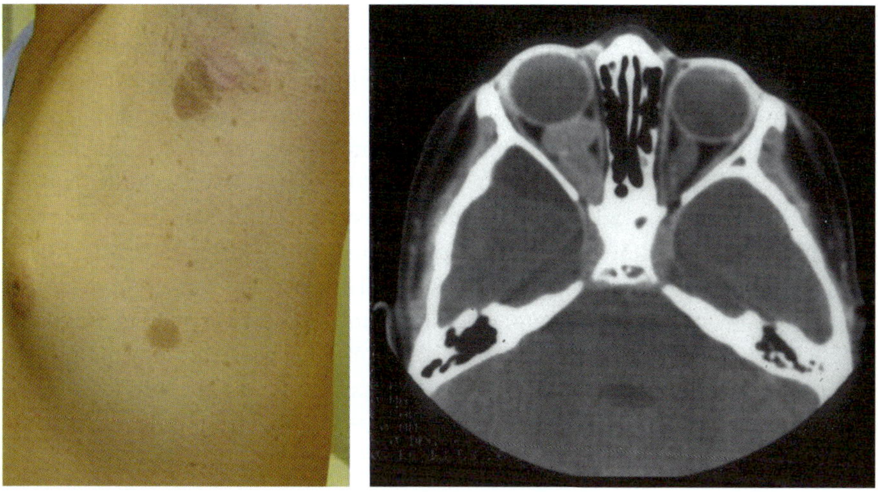

(a) (b)

Figure 2. Neurofibromatosis 1. (a) *Café-au-lait* patches and axillary freckling. (b) Optic glioma (arrow). Published in *Pediatr Clin North Am*, 39, ES Roach, Neurocutaneous syndromes, 591–620, Copyright Elsevier (1992).

diagnostic criteria for NF-1, usually by age 6 years. Inguinal and axillary freckling (Crowe sign) becomes evident during preschool years, and neurofibromas begin to develop in adolescence.

Although most of the tumors associated with NF-1 are benign neurofibromas or optic gliomas (Figure 2b), the potential for malignant transformation reduces the average life span by approximately 10 years. Systemic hypertension is more prevalent than in the general population; and this may be independent of the presence of pheochromocytoma or dysplastic arteries. NF-1 is associated with moyamoya syndrome, increasing the risk for stroke. Aqueductal stenosis is more common than in the general population. Short stature and macrocephaly are more common as well. Intelligence can be normal, but there is greater potential for mental retardation and behavioral concerns. Location and size of neurofibromas determine the associated symptoms.

Evaluations of individuals with neurofibromatosis 1

The individual with NF-1 warrants monitoring for development of optic gliomas, malignant transformation of cutaneous and noncutaneous neurofibromas and evolution of neurological symptoms related to growth of benign tumors. An ophthalmology evaluation at the time of diagnosis should establish whether

Lisch nodules are present and provide a baseline visual assessment. An MRI of the brain will help identify an optic glioma in children under the age of 5 years who are at greatest risk of developing gliomas, less cooperative with the ophthalmologic examination, and less forthcoming about subtle impairments in vision. In older individuals, neurological symptoms — headaches, seizures, change in personality or cognition, vision changes, and focal deficits — can guide requests for MRIs of the brain and orbits. Symptoms referable to the spinal cord warrant evaluation with neuroimaging of the spinal cord. Neuropsychological testing is helpful for appropriate classroom setting and placement. All these symptoms are best established and followed up on at least an annual basis by a neurologist, geneticist, or dedicated primary care provider. Molecular genetic testing in the form of genomic DNA and mitochondrial RNA analysis is utilized rarely in individuals with atypical features and in identifying a disease-causing mutation that can be transmitted to other children.

Neurofibromatosis 2

Neurofibromatosis 2 (NF-2) manifests primarily with tumors of the central nervous system and affects 1 in 35,000 to 50,000. NF-2 has autosomal dominant inheritance. The gene on chromosome 22 codes for schwannomin, a tumor suppressor. Schwannomin also is known as merlin: moesin-ezrin-radixin-like gene. Cutaneous stigmata are less impressive than in NF-1, and the primary ophthalmologic finding is presenile posterior subcapsular cataracts. Vestibular schwannomas, also known as acoustic neuromas, are the most common tumors; the presence of these tumors bilaterally is diagnostic of NF-2 (Figure 3.) Schwannomas involving other cranial nerves, ependymomas, meningiomas, and astrocytomas occur with higher frequency than in the general population. NF-2 presents relatively late compared to other neurocutaneous syndromes. Many patients may go undiagnosed. Earliest symptoms usually present in adolescence or early adulthood as hearing loss or tinnitus. Other presenting symptoms can include vertigo, facial weakness, ataxia and headache. Unilateral hearing loss is relatively common in the early stages even with evidence of bilateral vestibular schwannomas.

Evaluation of an individual with neurofibromatosis 2

Consider screening with annual auditory brainstem responses or brain MRI. At diagnosis, radiological evaluation of the entire neuroaxis with an MRI may help detect occult tumors. Thereafter, radiological evaluation of the spinal cord can be done on an as-needed basis. Molecular genetic testing is available but somatic mosaicism makes testing less sensitive.

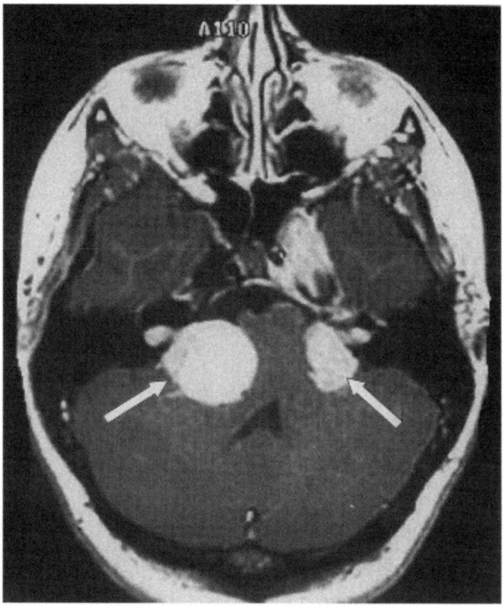

Figure 3. Vestibular schwannomas (arrows) in neurofibromatosis 2.

Sturge Weber Syndrome

The characteristic features of Sturge Weber syndrome (SWS) are a port-wine stain (Figure 4) and an associated angioma in the ipsilateral leptomeninges and brain. The nevus is a facial cutaneous angioma and typically involves the forehead or upper eyelid, but it may also involve both sides of the face and extend onto the trunk and limbs. Only about 20% of the individuals with a typical port-wine nevus have the leptomeningeal lesion or the resulting neurological dysfunction which lead to the diagnosis of SWS. Most of the individuals with SWS develop epilepsy. Other findings may include mental retardation, contralateral hemiparesis and hemiatrophy, and homonymous hemianopia. However, the clinical features are variable and patients may exhibit cutaneous lesions and seizures but with normal intelligence and no focal neurological deficits. Nevi that involve only the trunk or facial nevi that spare the upper face are rarely associated with intracranial angioma. Unlike most other neurocutaneous syndromes, SWS occurs sporadically and in all races.

Patients with Sturge Weber syndrome are at substantial risk of glaucoma with peak incidence during infancy and then again late in childhood. Seizures often occur early and herald hemiparesis that may be transient and then become permanent. Mental retardation is also common, especially in children with

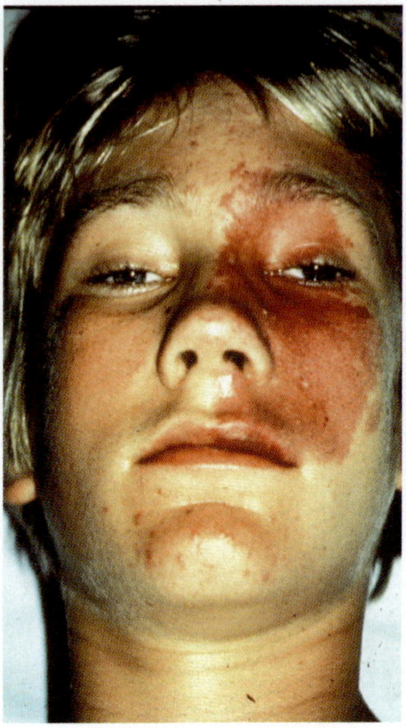

Figure 4. Port-wine stain in Sturge Weber syndrome.

evidence of bilateral intracranial involvement. Seizures, focal neurological deficits and cognitive impairment eventually stabilize.

Brain MRI is key in differentiating an isolated port-wine stain from SWS. Historically, skull X-rays and head CTs demonstrate tram-track calcifications outlining leptomeningeal angiomas; but these studies do not add to the information obtained from MRI. Functional neuroimaging such as PET and SPECT are useful for epilepsy surgery evaluation but are not recommended for other purposes. Similarly, cerebral arteriography is not required outside of mapping vasculature in individuals presenting for intracranial surgery. Hemispherectomy, or limited cortical resection for less extensive brain lesions are the surgical interventions of choice for patients with refractory epilepsy. Corpus callosotomy can lessen tonic or atonic seizures when the lesion is extensive. Given the risk of glaucoma, regular ophthalmologic evaluation with measurement of intraocular pressure is important.

Ataxia Telangiectasia

Ataxia telangiectasia (A-T) is an uncommon neurodegenerative disorder, affecting 1 in 40,000 to 1 in 100,000. Patients typically become symptomatic in early childhood with evidence of slowly progressive ataxia. Oculomotor apraxia is common although sometimes misidentified. Telangiectasias (dilated small blood vessels), immunodeficiency, and cellular sensitivity to ionizing radiation develop later. Distinctive skin lesions predominantly involve the sclerae, earlobes, and bridge of the nose. The combination of telangiectasias in a child with progressive ataxia is characteristic of A-T. A-T is an autosomal recessive disorder — unlike many of the inherited neurocutaneous syndromes. Ataxia telangiectasia mutated (ATM) is a protein kinase coded on chromosome 11, and it appears important in regulation of the cell cycle and protection against DNA damage. The gene frequency is as high as 1% in the general population. Unexplained ataxia in a child should raise suspicion for A-T, particularly if the ataxia is becoming progressively worse. The unsteadiness is typically truncal, affecting sitting as well as walking. Telangiectasias do not usually appear until 3 to 6 years of age, after the onset of ataxia.

The most striking non-neurological features of A-T are immune deficiencies. A dramatically increased risk for malignancy of the lymphoreticular system leads to a lymphoid malignancy by early adulthood in 10% to 15% of patients. The risk of non-lymphoid malignancy is also higher than in the general population. Frequent sinopulmonary infections, also related to immune deficiency, are common in patients with A-T. Serum α-fetoprotein and quantitative immunoglobulins often are performed at the time of diagnosis. Regular surveillance evaluation is key in the early diagnosis of malignancies. Cerebellar atrophy will appear on brain imaging that typically is performed in the evaluation of ataxia or abnormal eye movements. Undetectable or trace amounts of ATM protein by immunoblotting is the predominant means of confirming the diagnosis but radiosensitivity assays, chromosomal analysis and molecular gene testing also are available.

Von Hippel Lindau Disease

Von Hippel-Lindau (VHL) disease is characterized by hemangioblastomas in the retina and CNS as well as visceral cysts and tumors. Hemangioblastomas are benign, slow-growing vascular tumors that cause symptoms from hemorrhage or local mass effect. The most common manifestations of VHL are retinal and CNS hemangioblastomas and pancreatic cysts. Current prevalence estimates are approximately 1 in 40,000. VHL is an autosomal dominant disorder. The gene is a tumor suppressor on chromosome 3p that affects the function of hypoxia-induced factor, HIF2α. This regulation contributes to increased vascularization and upregulation of pro-angiogenic genes and other oxygen-sensitive genes via hypoxia response elements (HRE). These genes include vascular endothelial growth factor (VEGF), platelet-derived growth factor (PDGF), transforming growth factor alpha (TGFα), glucose transporter-1 (GLUT-1), carbonic anhydrase IX, and erythropoietin (EPO). In particular, VEGF is important in angiogenesis.

The initial symptoms of VHL usually arise from effects of the vascular anomalies in the CNS, most commonly the cerebellum. These may begin in the second decade of life and include: headache, ataxia, nausea and vomiting, and nystagmus. The symptoms are often intermittent or slowly progressive, but up to 20% of patients have an acute onset of symptoms following mild head trauma. Other common sites of hemangioblastomas are the spinal cord and medulla. Spinal hemangioblastomas typically present with sensory loss, weakness or focal back or neck pain. The incidence of cerebellar hemangioblastomas increases with age: 84% of patients have at least one by 60 years. Childhood onset of symptoms is unusual, but retinal hemangioblastomas may occur in children as young as 1 year. Some patients may present with pheochromocytoma or renal, pancreatic, hepatic, or epididymal tumors.

Renal cysts are present in more than half of individuals with VHL, although the patients may be asymptomatic. Extensive renal cysts rarely lead to renal failure. Of greater concern is renal cell carcinoma, which develops in more than 70% of patients and is the leading cause of death in patients with VHL. These tumors are usually multiple and tend to occur at a younger age than sporadic renal cell carcinoma. Pheochromocytomas occur in 7% to 19% of patients and may be the only clinical manifestation of VHL, even in carefully screened individuals. Even in the absence of hemorrhage, vision loss may occur. This is especially true, when large and centrally located retinal hemangioblastomas are present. Hemorrhage may lead to retinal injury and detachment, glaucoma, uveitis, macular edema, and sympathetic ophthalmitis. Endolymphatic sac tumors can also affect 10–15% of individuals with VHL. Sometimes they are bilateral. Presenting symptoms can be abrupt change in hearing accompanying hemorrhage or vertigo and tinnitus.

Hemangioblastomas are best seen with contrast-enhanced MRI of the brain and entire spinal cord. Routine screening of the brain should include thin sections through the posterior fossa. Arteriography is not necessary for diagnosis but is valuable in demonstrating the feeding vessels if surgical resection is planned. Careful screening is the most important aspect of management of VHL. The diagnosis is confirmed by molecular genetic testing. Screening is mandatory for all first-degree relatives in a family with VHL or pheochromocytoma. Other indications for clinical screening include pancreatic cysts, multiple or bilateral renal cell tumors, retinal hemangiomas, and cerebellar hemangioblastomas. Molecular analysis for the VHL gene reduces the number of asymptomatic relatives requiring surveillance; only relatives who have inherited the VHL mutation need annual screening.

References

Bodensteiner J, Roach ES. *Sturge-Weber Syndrome*, 2nd edn. Mt Freedom, NJ: Sturge-Weber Foundation, 2010.

Butman JA, Linehan WM, Lonser RR. Neurological manifestations of von Hippel-Lindau disease. *JAMA*. 2008.300:1334–1342.

Evans DG. Neurofibromatosis type 2. In: Roach ES., Miller VS. (eds.). *Neurocutaneous Syndromes*. London: Cambridge University Press. 2004. pp. 50–59.

Islam M. Roach ES. Neurocutaneous syndromes. In: Bradley W., Daroff R., Fenichel G., Jankovic J. (eds.). *Neurology in Clinical Practice*. Philadelphia: Butterworth Heinemann Elsevier, 2008. pp. 1821–1853.

16

IDIOPATHIC INTRACRANIAL HYPERTENSION

Shawn Aylward

A 12-year-old female is evaluated in the Emergency Department for the chief complaint of daily headache and blurred vision. The symptoms have been present for the past 3 weeks. The girl describes the pain as a pulsatile headache that is worse in the morning or any time she bends over. The patient's weight is > 95th percentile, while her height is in the 50th percentile. Fundoscopic examination reveals blurring of the optic discs' margins; the patient also has bilateral enlargement of the blind spot. With the above in mind, the patient underwent CT scan of the head. The test was deemed to be within normal limits. A lumbar puncture revealed the patient to have an opening pressure of 35 cm of water.

Introduction

Increased intracranial pressure was first described by Quincke in 1897 shortly after he introduced the concept of the lumbar puncture. The author reported patients with symptoms of increased intracranial pressure in the presence of unremarkable cerebrospinal fluid chemistry, and termed this condition "meningitis serosa." Over the years, idiopathic intracranial hypertension has been known by different names reflecting advancements in the practice of medicine. In 1904, the term "pseudotumor" cerebri was coined. This term reflected the fact that increased intracranial pressure presents with symptoms similar to those found in a patient

---

Division of Child Neurology, Nationwide Children's Hospital and The Ohio State University, Columbus, Ohio, USA

with an intracranial mass. In 1955, the condition was renamed benign intracranial hypertension to avoid the negative connotation associated with a "pseudo-cancer" diagnosis. In the 1980s, following a series of reports describing vision loss, the constellation of signs and symptoms was renamed idiopathic intracranial hypertension (IIH).

When asked to recount the usual patient with IIH, most physicians will describe an obese, middle-aged woman, of childbearing age, complaining of headaches and blurred vision. And although this is the most common patient illustration, IIH is seen in all age groups and in both genders. In the United States, the annual incidence of IIH is estimated at 0.9 per 100,000. As indicated above, IIH is more common in females (3.5 per 100,000) and even more frequent in obese females (12–19 per 100,000). The female to male ratio has been reported to be approximately 4:1. More recently, the diagnosis of IIH is being made in younger patients. This trend likely reflects either the increasing problem of childhood obesity, or increased awareness of the condition. The former issues set aside, the authors of recent reports have indicated that pre-pubertal patients with IIH are usually not obese and that both genders are equally affected. In the aforementioned studies, however, the definition of pre- vs. post-pubertal is often made by age rather than by the presence of secondary sexual characteristics, so the conclusions reached may not be as accurate.

There are no pediatric-specific criteria for the diagnosis of IIH. Thus, clinicians use the modified version of Dandy's criteria which were intended for adult patients. Dandy stipulated that a patient with IIH must have:

1. Signs and symptoms of increased intracranial pressure.
2. Non-focal neurological examination (with the exception of cranial nerve palsy).
3. Elevated cerebrospinal fluid pressure (>25 cm of H_2O), with unremarkable CSF chemical analysis.
4. Exclusion of other causes of IIH such as a mass lesion, hydrocephalus, or vascular malformation via imaging studies.

The exact cause of increased intracranial pressure remains elusive. Current consensus is that the condition is a result of impaired CSF absorption. But there is no agreement on what impairs CSF absorption. One school of thought points to reduced CSF absorption at the level of the arachnoid villi as a consequence of increased protein in the CSF, a history of a prior infection, hemorrhage, or possibly the compounding results of increased pressure progressively compressing the villi. The second school of thought postulates that impaired absorption is the result of increased CSF flow resistance from raised venous pressure secondary to venous outflow obstruction. It is suspected that a genetic predisposition to IIH exists. If such is the case, it is likely the result of a "multi-hit" phenomenon, as the condition rarely has a consistent familial inheritance pattern.

Clinical Presentation

The patient with IIH presents with a history of recent onset daily, pulsatile, frontal headaches. These are often worse when lying down or in the morning. Maneuvers that increase intracranial pressure such as coughing, Valsalva maneuver, or bending over can worsen the symptoms. Patients who have severe optic nerve edema often report exacerbation of the headache with eye movements. The cause of this phenomenon is likely related to slight traction on the swollen and distended optic nerves. Other common symptoms include tinnitus (often described as a whooshing or ringing sound), blurred vision, transient visual obscurations, and neck stiffness. Less frequent symptoms include vertigo, nausea, and emesis. The patient's physical examination should not make evident any neurological deficits with the occasional exception of cranial nerve palsies. Sixth-nerve palsy is the most common followed by third-, fourth-, seventh- or twelfth-cranial-nerve palsy. The abducens nerve is more vulnerable due to downward displacement of the brain from the increased pressure; this in turn presses the nerve against the petrous temporal ridge.

Symptoms of IIH are not exclusive to the condition. Therefore, IIH should be a diagnosis of exclusion; even if the patient has some of the common risk factors and an elevated opening pressure on lumbar puncture. The authors of several reports have associated IIH to a variety of systemic diseases. Many of these are case reports or small patient-series with conflicting results. The only predisposing factors that have been decisively linked to IIH are: obesity, especially of recent onset and with rapid weight gain, post-pubertal patient, and female gender. A list of the conditions frequently associated to IIH is presented in Table 1. Similarly, a list of medications that have been associated with development of IIH is presented in Table 2.

Some conditions clearly lead to secondary intracranial hypertension. Therefore, the term *idiopathic* intracranial hypertension would be inaccurate. Instead, the patient should be diagnosed with "intracranial hypertension secondary to . . . ." An example would be the patient with intracranial hypertension secondary to a glioblastoma multiforme. Other examples are listed in Table 3.

Diagonsis

Since the symptoms of IIH are not specific to the disorder, other causes that may mimic IIH should be ruled out. A thorough review of the patient's medical history should be performed. This will help uncover potential endocrine, infectious,

Table 1. Disorders associated with increased risk of IIH.

- Obesity (especially recent and significant weight gain)
- Iron deficiency anemia
- Hypoparathyroidism
- Hyperthyroidism
- Early in correction of hypothyroidism
- Sarcoidosis
- Addison disease
- Systemic Lupus
- Prothrombotic states — Lupus, Behcet and Crohn disease
- Kidney transplant (treated with high dose corticosteroids)
- Impaired renal function (receiving growth hormones)
- Leukemia
- Lymphoma
- Vitamin A (intoxication and deficiency)
- Vitamin D deficiency
- Pregnancy
- Irregular menses
- Polycystic ovarian syndrome
- Hypertension
- Chronic otitis or sinusitis
- AVM
- Recent varicella infection
- Lyme disease**
- Trauma (usually with venous sinus thrombosis)
- Refeeding syndrome following prolonged starvation

**Lyme disease is debated as a predisposing factor as in theory, the CSF will be abnormal, and by the Dandy criteria, would not fit IIH.

traumatic, medication, and oncological causes. Laboratory studies should include: complete blood count, complete metabolic panel, thyroid panel, and vitamin A level. Thrombotic and thrombophilic profiles, erythrocyte sedimentation rate, angiotensin converting enzymes, vitamin D level, and anti-nuclear antibodies should be included when appropriate.

A fundoscopic examination should be done by an experienced clinician, preferably an ophthalmologist. The true definition of papilledema is the presence of optic disc edema in the setting of increased intracranial pressure. In the absence of documented intracranial hypertension, the correct terminology for a swollen optic nerve head is disc edema or disc swelling. The presence of venous pulsations is a good indicator against the diagnosis of optic nerve edema. However, their absence is not necessarily diagnostic of edema. Bilateral papilledema is seen in

Table 2. Drugs associated with increased risk of IIH.

- Tetracycline*
- Minocycline
- Vitamin A
- Growth hormone
- Insulin growth-factor I
- Oral contraceptives
- Lithium
- Levothyroxine
- Cytarabine
- All-trans retinoic acid (especially children under 8)
- Corticosteroids (current or withdrawal (including tapers))
- Accutane (isotretinoin)
- Trimethoprim-sulfamethoxizole

*It is believed that tetracyclines impair CSF absorption at the arachnoid villi by affecting the function of cyclic adenosine monophosphate.

Table 3. IIH mimickers — Conditions that can cause symptoms also seen in IIH.

- Infectious — meningitis (bacterial, viral, chemical), encephalitis, brain abscess, Lyme disease
- Trauma — epidural, subdural and subarachnoid hematoma, cerebral contusion, and edema
- Intracranial mass — tumor, lymphoma, arteriovenous malformation, cavernous hemagioma
- Intracranial hemorrhage — intracerebral and intraventricular
- Headache syndromes — migraine, tension headache medication overuse headache
- Ischemic stroke
- Hydrocephalus
- Venous sinus thrombosis
- Hypoxic conditions — airway obstruction, hypoventilation, obstructive sleep apnea

nearly all patients with IIH, although there are often subtle differences in the degree of edema. In the setting of unilateral edema, an effort should be made to find alternative causes for the patient's symptoms. Ultrasound of the optic nerves can rule out other causes of pseudo-papilledema such as drusen, or tilted optic

Table 4. Differential diagnosis for optic nerve edema.

- IIH
- Pseuodpapilledema — drusen
- Tilted optic discs
- Anomalous branching or tortuous optic vessels
- Congenital optic abnormalities
- Optic neuritis
- Anterior ischemic optic neuropathy

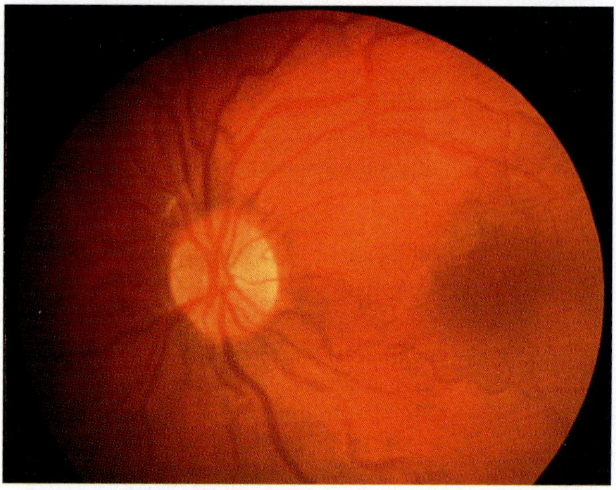

Figure 1. Normal optic disc.

discs (see Table 4). Goldman's kinetic perimetry or Humphrey's automated static perimetry should be used to monitor for visual field deficits, which is often subtle. Visual loss usually begins with enlargement of the physiologic blind spot together with inferonasal visual deficits on visual field testing. By the time a patient reports decrease in peripheral vision, injury to the optic nerve is apt to be permanent. Except in extreme cases, the severity of the visual field deficit does not correlate with either the severity of the edema or the cerebrospinal fluid pressure.

The degree of papilledema is graded with the Frisen scale assigning a value of 0–4 (see Figures 1–5). Grade 0 indicates minimal nasal edema. With grade 1, edema involves a C-shaped distribution sparing the temporal side. Grade 2 edema involves 360 degrees of the optic nerve. Blurring of the vessels as they cross over the disc margin represents grade 3 edema. With grade 4 edema, all vascular markings

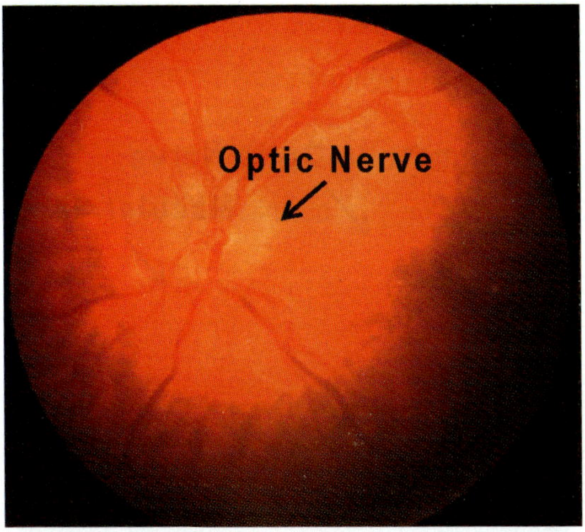

Figure 2. Mild optic nerve edema (grade 1+).

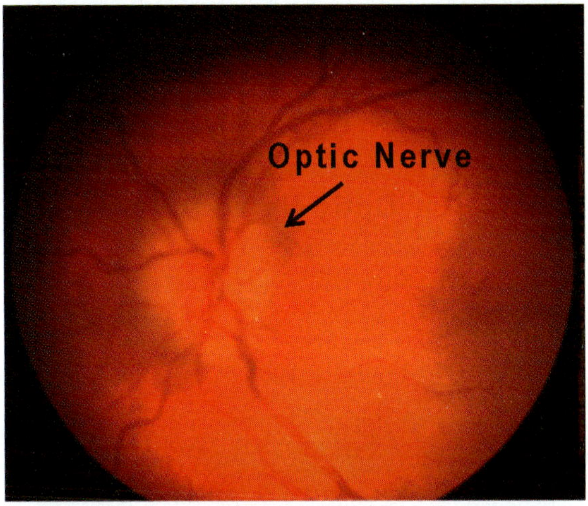

Figure 3. Moderate optic nerve edema (grade 3+).

around the optic nerve as well as the optic disc itself are lost. Evidence of edema of the retina surrounding the disc in the form of hemorrhages or even a macular star can be observer.

All patients with suspected IIH require a lumbar puncture to document the opening pressure. Due to the possibility of an intracranial mass, it is recommended

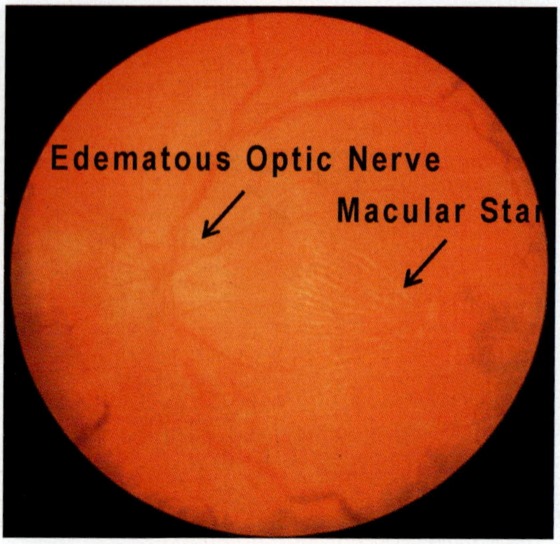

Figure 4. Severe edema with macular star (grade 4+).

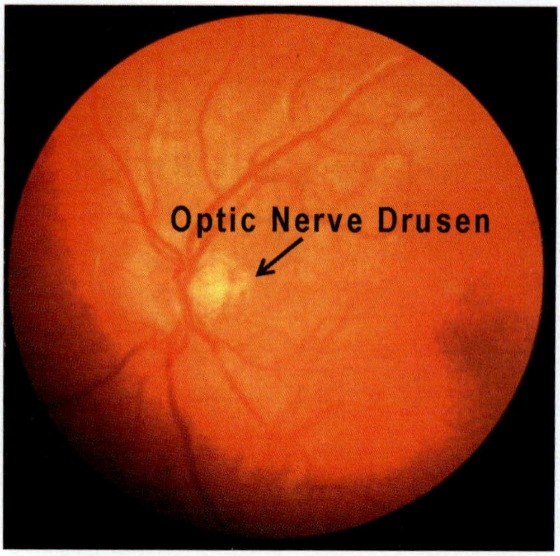

Figure 5. Optic disc drusen.

that prior to the procedure, all patients undergo CT scan of the head or MRI of the brain. For the lumbar puncture, the patient should be placed in the left lateral decubitus position; the opening pressure should never be obtained while the patient is sitting up. The use of interventional radiology techniques may be required when adequate anatomic landmarks are not palpable. Standard patient positioning is with the legs and neck extended. Avery *et al.* performed a small study comparing pressure readings when the patient's legs and neck were flexed vs. when they were extended. Analysis of their results revealed a minimal pressure change, around 5 cm of water, between the two positions. Although the authors advocated not altering the patient's position to obtain pressure readings, convention dictates that the pressure be measured when the patient's legs and neck are extended. Hypoventilation associated with the sedated patient can artificially raise the intracranial pressure. Conversely, hyperventilation can cause a hypocarbic state and lower the pressure.

Currently accepted standards are that the normal opening pressure for an adult is <20 cm H_2O. IIH is diagnosed in patients whose opening pressure is >25 cm H_2O. The 20–25 cm H_2O range is of unclear clinical significance. In a recent editorial, Avery *et al.* recorded the opening pressure in a series of children undergoing lumbar puncture. The authors suggest that, in the pediatric population, pressures over 28 cm of H_2O should be considered abnormal. Unfortunately, their population size was too small to alter the current standards. If the opening pressure is found to be elevated, attempts should be made to remove enough fluid to return the pressure to the normal range. The closing pressure should always be documented. Cerebrospinal fluid analysis such as glucose, protein, cell count, and bacterial cultures are routinely ordered. Viral cultures, arbovirus, EBV, CMV, HSV, and Lyme PCR can be added if supported by the clinical scenario. As mentioned above, to fulfill Dandy's criteria, the CSF analysis should be unremarkable. A mild pleocytosis, however, is not uncommon. To reduce the possibility of post-lumbar puncture intracranial hypotension, the patient should remain in a horizontal position for 1 hour after the procedure.

In addition to MRI of the brain, the evaluation of a patient with IIH should include magnetic resonance angiography and magnetic resonance venography. These studies will help rule out blood vessel malformations and thrombosis as causes of the intracranial hypertension. In a small subset of patients, MRI of the brain may reveal subtle findings of IIH. These include: lateral venous sinus stenosis, empty sella sign, slit-like ventricles, flattening of the posterior aspect of the globe, or optic nerve edema (bulging of the optic nerve head, or frank swelling of the nerve). The above mentioned venous sinus stenosis, is thought to be secondary to the increased pressure and not its cause. The authors of several studies have reported that repeating the MR venography immediately after removing a large volume of cerebrospinal fluid may reveal resolution of the stenosis.

Treatment

Ideally, a multidisciplinary team addresses the needs of a patient with IIH. That team consists of a neurologist, ophthalmologist, neurosurgeon, dietician, physical therapist, and psychologist. Unfortunately, treatment recommendations are largely based on anecdotal information. Few retrospective or unblinded studies on the management of IIH have been completed. Regardless of treatment modality used, a patient with IIH should have close ophthalmologic follow-up with repeated fundoscopic and visual field evaluations. A common schedule for ophthalmologic follow-up is 1, 3, and 6 months following diagnosis and initiation of treatment.

Lumbar punctures can temporally improve the subjective symptoms of IIH. Prior to the use of medications in the management for IIH, treatment consisted of serial lumbar punctures — sometimes twice a day. Owing to the fact that the lumbar puncture does little to alter the production rate of CSF, the repeated lumbar punctures likely caused enough local trauma to allow for a residual cerebrospinal fluid leak. Since serial lumbar punctures carry significant discomfort and morbidity, and that similar or better results are obtained with medications, this practice has become obsolete.

Pharmacological treatment of IIH

The most commonly used medication for the treatment of IIH is acetazolamide. This medication acts through carbonic anhydrase inhibition, decreasing cerebrospinal fluid production by lowering the transport of sodium across the choroidal epithelium. For children, a recommended dose is 25 mg/kg/day divided twice a day. In adolescents, the dose used is 0.5–1 g/day divided twice a day. The target dose in pediatrics patients is 1–2 g divided twice a day; 3–4 g divided twice a day can be used in adolescents and adults. Patients may complain of food having a metallic taste, especially carbonated beverages. This side effect often leads to transient anorexia, which aides with weight lost (please see below). Patients can notice paresthesias in distal segments of the extremities and the perioral region. These symptoms are most common when initiating treatment or when the dose is increased and they are usually transient. Increasing the intake of potassium rich foods such as orange juice and bananas reduces the severity of this discomfort. Nephrolithiasis is a rare but serious complication of the use of acetazolamide. Any patient complaining of blood in the urine, unexplained fever, or back pain should be screened for kidney stones. Metabolic acidosis is also rare; it should be monitored through a renal panel 4–6 weeks after starting treatment with acetazolamide. Finally, aplastic anemia has been reported to occur in patients taking acetazolamide. Fortunately, the risk is very low and routine monitoring is not necessary.

Furosemide and topiramate have been used in patients unable to tolerate acetazolamide. Both medications have been shown to be as effective as acetazolamide. Furosemide works by increasing diuresis and reducing sodium transport into the brain. The usual dose is 1–2 mg/kg/day divided into 2–3 doses. In adolescents and adults, an appropriate dose is 40–120 mg two to three times a day. Serum electrolytes should be monitored closely and potassium supplementation given as needed. The authors of several studies suggest an added benefit when furosemide is used in conjunction with acetazolamide. Topiramate is a medication known to have weak carbonic anhydrase inhibition properties. It is hypothesized that topiramate's mode of action is similar to that of acetazolamide. As such, the same side effects can occur and monitoring should be similar to patients taking acetazolamide. Topiramate, however, has other side effects such as anhydrosis, mild word finding difficulties, and it is a more potent appetite suppressant. The most serious side effect of topiramate is development of acute angle-closure glaucoma. This, fortunately, is rarely seen in the pediatric population. Owing to numerous side effects including weight gain, corticosteroids are no longer routinely used to treat IIH. A situation where steroids might be of use is to stabilize a patient whose vision is rapidly deteriorating and who is not responding to standard pharmacological therapy.

Intravenous methylprednisolone is given at 15 mg/kg. The typical oral prednisone dosing is 2 mg/kg/day for two weeks. This is then followed by a two-week taper as sudden cessation of steroids can lead to rebound increased intracranial pressure and symptom worsening.

Weight control

For obese patients, referral to a pediatric weight loss program is strongly advised. The authors of several studies have shown that, except for discontinuation of offending medications, weight loss is the single most important intervention that may reverse IIH and avoid its reccurrence. Rapid, massive weight loss is discouraged. Rather, slow steady weight loss is recommended. The patient should be given an attainable goal of 2 lbs. per month. Patients should be frequently reminded that weight loss is not a short-term process, but rather a life-long and lifestyle change. A dietitian can aid the patient make healthy food choices and select proper portion sizes. The dietitian will also help monitor the patient's weight and modify the program as the patient progresses. Physical trainers or physical therapists can help the patient develop an exercise routine that fits their level of conditioning. Involvement of a psychologist also improves the potential of a successful weight loss program. Occasionally, morbidly obese patients may wish to pursue bariatric surgery to assist with weight loss. This option needs to be evaluated in a case-by-case basis, and the conversation should always include the surgeon.

Surgical interventions

Despite the pharmacological treatments available, some patients will experience worsening symptoms, even on maximal therapy. Optic-nerve-sheath fenestration decreases the pressure on the optic nerve head preventing further injury. The procedure consists of a series of slits along the nerve sheath. Complications are rare and include ischemic optic neuropathy, transient blindness, pupillary midriasis due to sympathetic ganglion injury, and retrobulbar hemorrhage. It is unclear precisely how this intervention works. It is thought to cause scarring of the arachnoid around the optic nerve isolating the disk from the increased cerebrospinal fluid pressure. Fenestration can even be effective when done unilaterally, with resolution of papilledema even in the nonoperated eye.

Lumbo- and ventriculo-peritoneal shunts lower the intracranial pressure, thus improving the pain component of IIH. Lumbo-peritoneal shunts have a high failure rate, often requiring multiple revisions. These shunts are associated with an over-shunting phenomenon and acquired Arnold-Chiari malformation type 1. Ventriculo-peritoneal shunts fail less frequently than lumbo-peritoneal shunts. Some surgeons shy away from placing ventriculo-peritoneal shunts in patients with IIH as many have normal or small ventricles. The use of endoscopic shunt placement has made the procedure more successful. Risks associated with shunt placement include infection, abdominal pain, and migration of the peritoneal catheter.

Emergent surgery should be considered in patients at risk for acute vision loss. This would include those patients with severe visual deficits at the time of presentation, severe papilledema (especially in patients where reliable vision field testing is difficult), and progressive visual lost despite maximizing pharmacological therapy.

Outcome

Pain and permanent visual loss are the two major complications of IIH. By the time IIH is diagnosed, up to 20% of patients will already have some documented loss of visual acuity. Fortunately, this is permanent in only 10% of those patients. Pubertal or post-pubertal children tend to fair worse than pre-pubertal children. Resolution of papilledema will often take 3–6 months following treatment initiation. There is no consensus on treatment duration; although it is commonly continued for 4–6 months after clinical and symptomatic relief. Some practitioners opt to repeat a lumbar puncture to document pressure normalization prior to weaning the medication off and again 4–6 weeks after medications have been discontinued. Most practitioners use the return of symptoms, including papilledema, to guide the management. Recurrence of IIH is reported in 10–20% of patients. Recurrence is more common in those who have failed to reduce or maintain their goal weight. It is common for IIH patients to develop migraine or other headache syndromes following resolution of the IIH. In those cases, patients benefit from standard headache prophylaxis.

References

Avery RA, Mistry RD, Shah SS, *et al.* Patient position during lumbar puncture has no meaningful effect on cerebrospinal fluid opening pressure in children. *J Child Neurol.* 2010.25:616–619.

Avery RA, Shah SS, Licht DJ, *et al.* Reference range for cerebrospinal fluid opening pressure in children. *N Engl J Med.* 2010.363:891–893.

Rangwala LM, Liu GT. Pediatric idiopathic intracranial hypertension. *Surv Ophthalmol.* 2007.52:597–617.

Schexnayder LKC, *et al.* Presentation, investigation and management of idiopathic intracranial hypertension in children. *Curr Paediatr.* 2006.16:336–341.

Smith JL. Whence pseudotumor cerebri? *J Clin Neuroophthalmol.* 1985.5:55–56.

17

SYNCOPE

Shane F. Tsai, Jack R. Stines and Timothy M. Hoffman

A 15-year-old girl presents for evaluation of multiple episodes of "passing out spells" within the past year. The first episode occurred while taking a hot shower. Following the event, the child had an evident scalp hematoma. The next incident happened after standing up from her desk at school. Evaluation by the specialist was prompted by her losing consciousness during a cross country race. The child indicated that at the end of the competition, she became lightheaded and describes seeing "spots" in her field of vision before passing out. According to witnesses, she exhibited mild jerking of her arms but no incontinence of bowel or bladder. She was responsive after a few minutes, but complained of fatigue. The review of systems is significant for occasional dizziness when arising from a seated to standing position. The symptoms subside if she sits down quickly. The patient drinks fluids throughout the day, and carries a water bottle when she runs. She occasionally drinks caffeinated beverages. Past medical history is unremarkable, and the patient does not take medications regularly. Family medical history is significant for: a paternal uncle with "cardiac" health issues; the maternal grandfather dying unexpectedly in the sixth decade of life; and a cousin who passed away following a drowning accident. On physical examination, the patient has normal body habitus and vital signs. Orthostatic blood pressure measurements are normal. Focused cardiovascular examination revealed: normal heart sounds, and a soft systolic flow murmur. Peripheral pulses are strong and symmetric, and there is no appreciable radial-femoral delay.

Division of Pediatric Cardiology, Nationwide Children's Hospital and The Ohio State University, Columbus, Ohio, USA

Highlights

The case described is consistent with the diagnosis of vasodepressor syncope, a common non–life-threatening diagnosis. However, there are several potential red flags in this case which should be recognized.

- Exercise-associated syncope is concerning for potential life-threatening conditions, including structural heart disease, cardiomyopathy, or arrhythmia.
- Serious injuries sustained during the syncopal episodes suggest absence of a sufficient prodrome to avert loss of consciousness, and may be related to ventricular arrhythmia.
- Neurological seizure must be distinguished from "seizure-like" activities which result from cerebral hypoxia associated with neurocardiogenic syncope.
- Cardiac-related death in the family history, including congestive heart failure and myocardial infarction, must be distinguished from sudden cardiac death related to a hereditary condition. Unexplained drowning is suggestive of a channelopathy.
- Benign murmurs of childhood and adolescence are common, and should not be confused with pathological murmurs associated with structural heart disease.

Therefore, the examiner is expected to obtain an in-depth case history and perform a detailed physical exam in order to distinguish benign from potentially lethal conditions; ones that would warrant further investigation.

Syncope is the transient loss of consciousness and postural tone secondary to a decrease in cerebral blood flow and oxygenation. In children and adolescents, it is most often benign; but it causes significant anxiety in patients and their families. Approximately 15% of pediatric patients will experience an episode of syncope prior to the end of adolescence. The peak incidence is between 15 and 19 years of age, and it is more common in females than males.

Differential Diagnosis of Syncope

Common benign

(1) *Neurocardiogenic (vasovagal) syncope* is the most common form of syncope in the pediatric population. In susceptible individuals, the most likely mechanism is pooling of blood in the peripheral vasculature with a subsequent decrease in systemic venous return. This results in vigorous ventricular contractions and subsequent paradoxical cardioinhibitory and vasodilatory response from the central nervous system, which in turn causes bradycardia and hypotension.

Neurocardiogenic syncope can be provoked by prolonged standing, rising quickly from a lying or seated position, crowded rooms, emotional distress, pain, or vigorous exercise in warm conditions. Presyncopal symptoms may occur well before loss of consciousness. These include light-headedness, dizziness, visual changes, headache, nausea, and diaphoresis. Injury is usually avoided as a consequence of the "warning" or prodrome. Loss of consciousness is transient, and patients quickly return to their normal state of alertness. There may be brief "seizure-like" activity associated with the event, but there is no post-ictal period — a feature that distinguishes syncope from a seizure. Situational syncope is another form of neurally mediated syncope with a similar mechanism. This form of syncope may be triggered by micturation, coughing, defecation, swallowing, or by the extension of the neck while combing or blow drying hair.

(2) *Breath holding spells* are common in infants and children, and typically occur between the ages of 6 months to 6 years. Most children experience the first episode prior to 18 months of age. Spells follow a typical pattern; one that is prompted by pain or anger. The child will hold his or her breath, and then become cyanotic or extremely pale. There is severely decreased muscle tone and subsequent loss of consciousness; these may be accompanied by brief tonic-clonic activity. The child quickly recovers consciousness. Parents should be informed of the benign nature of these episodes. Some authors, however, have reported an association between breath holding spells and iron deficiency anemia. Thus, individuals should be screened as appropriate.

Structural heart disease

(1) *Hypertrophic cardiomyopathy* (*HCM*) is an autosomal dominant condition affecting the cardiac sarcomere. It is characterized by thickening of the left ventricle without chamber dilation. HCM is the most common cause of sudden death in the young. Volume depletion leads to decreased stroke volume and potential increase in left ventricular outflow tract gradient. Hypotension and syncope may result from inadequate cardiac output. Avoidance of intense exertion and athletic competition is usually recommended. Patients with unexplained syncope are at high risk of sudden death, and should be evaluated urgently.

(2) *Anomalous coronary arteries* encompass a rare group of malformations that may occur in isolation or may be associated with congenital heart disease. The most common anomaly is where the right coronary artery originates from the left sinus of Valsalva. Patients may present with syncope, chest pain, or sudden cardiac death during exercise. Myocardial ischemia results from compression of an interarterial

coronary artery between the aorta and pulmonary artery. Syncope or chest pain brings this diagnosis to mind.

(3) *Congenital heart disease* may be complicated by syncope, although neurally mediated episodes remain the most common cause. There are few structural congenital abnormalities which may cause syncope. Similar to hypertrophic cardiomyopathy, left ventricular outflow tract obstruction may occur with aortic stenosis. However, children with aortic stenosis are typically asymptomatic unless the stenosis is severe. Significant ventricular dysfunction and heart failure associated with complex congenital abnormalities may increase the risk of syncope. Patients with moderate to severe pulmonary hypertension, whether primary or secondary, are also at risk.

(4) *Arrhythmogenic right ventricular cardiomyopathy* (*ARVC*) is an autosomal dominant disorder with variable penetrance and expression; it is associated with a genetic defect of desmosomal proteins. ARVC is characterized by fibrofatty replacement of the ventricular myocardium and is associated with arrhythmias originating from the right ventricle. Initial presentation includes syncope or sudden death. Syncope and ventricular arrhythmias are usually exercise related.

(5) *Acute myocarditis* is an inflammatory process characterized by infiltration of the myocardium with resulting necrosis. Viral infections, including coxsackievirus, adenovirus, enterovirus, and parvovirus B19, are the most common etiology. Syncope may occur from ventricular hypokinesis and significantly reduced cardiac output.

(6) *Dilated cardiomyopathy* has multiple potential etiologies, and is characterized by cardiac dilation and decreased systolic function. Pathogenesis includes infectious, metabolic, toxic, ischemic, and hereditary factors. In children, the primary cause often remains undiagnosed. Symptoms of congestive heart failure may develop gradually. Syncope may be caused by atrial or ventricular arrhythmias, atrioventricular conduction defect, or low cardiac output. Syncope is associated with a high risk of sudden death.

Primary arrhythmia

(1) *Supraventricular tachycardia* (*SVT*) is a relatively frequent occurring arrhythmia, but rarely the cause of syncope. That said, SVT-caused syncope is associated with sinus nodal dysfunction and prolonged sinus pause at the termination of tachycardia. These abnormalities result in loss of consciousness. In other cases, the tachycardia may trigger a vasodepressor response which produces syncope.

Particular note should be made of patients with evidence of ventricular pre-excitation.

(2) *Wolff-Parkinson–White syndrome* (*WPW*) is characterized by the presence of an accessory pathway for the depolarizing current. This abnormality is made evident by the presence of a delta wave on the electrocardiogram. Atrial fibrillation is the presenting arrhythmia in up to 20% of patients with WPW, and rapid conduction via the bypass tract can result in hemodynamic instability. In rare instances, the conduction anomaly can lead to ventricular fibrillation and sudden death.

(3) *Long QT syndrome*, or prolongation of the QT interval, may be congenital or acquired. Syncope is associated with ventricular arrhythmia, and may result in sudden death. Family history of congenital deafness is suggestive of *Jervell and Lange–Nielsen syndrome*, an autosomal recessive condition associated with sudden death. *Romano–Ward syndrome* is not associated with deafness, and is transmitted in autosomal dominant fashion. Acquired prolongation may be caused by multiple etiologies. Careful attention should be paid to prescription drug use, including antimicrobial and antifungal agents, antidepressants, and antipsychotics. Antiarrhythmic drugs may paradoxically be pro-arrhythmic, including Vaughn-Williams Class IA, IC, and III agents. Electrolyte disturbances, including hypocalcemia, hypokalemia, and hypomagnesemia, can all prolong repolarization. Other potential causes of QT prolongation include myocarditis, head injury or cerebrovascular accident, and ventricular conduction disturbances (bundle branch block, pre-excitation).

(4) *Catecholaminergic polymorphic ventricular tachycardia* is an electrically unstable rhythm characterized by bidirectional or continuously varying (polymorphic) QRS morphology, and ventricular rates of greater than 200 beats per minute. It typically occurs in childhood or adolescence and in the absence of structural heart disease. Patients present with life-threatening ventricular arrhythmia associated with emotional or physical stress. Gene mutations have been identified in the cardiac ryanodine receptor and calsequestrin 2.

(5) *Brugada syndrome* is a channelopathy inherited in autosomal dominant manner. Gene mutations in the sodium channel SCN5A have been linked to the illness. Brugada syndrome is characterized by sudden death associated with one of several distinguishing electrocardiogram patterns (please see "Diagnostic tests"). Patients are prone to develop ventricular tachyarrhythmias that lead to syncope, cardiac arrest, or sudden death. It most commonly affects healthy men between ages 30 and 50 years. In children, arrhythmia may be more likely during a febrile

illness. It may also be unmasked by other clinical conditions, including alcohol intoxication, hyper- or hypokalemia, and hypercalcemia.

(6) *Postural tachycardia syndrome* is orthostatic intolerance in response to postural changes. Patients experience an exaggerated increase in heart rate without change in blood pressure. Females are affected 5:1 compared to males. Symptoms include lightheadedness, dizziness, and fatigue. Syncope, however, is uncommon.

(7) *Short QT syndrome* is a rare condition characterized by a very short corrected QT interval (less than 0.30 seconds); it is transmitted in an autosomal dominant pattern. Short QT syndrome is associated with atrial fibrillation, as well as ventricular tachycardia and vetricular fibrillation. Symptoms include palpitations and syncope; sudden death may occur at any age.

Miscellaneous

Seizures should be considered in the differential diagnosis of syncope. Patients with true seizures are more likely to have an aura, prolonged tonic-clonic activity, and a postictal phase. The authors of several studies, however, have demonstrated that some patients with "typical seizures" in fact have cardiac-related disorders. This possibility should be considered in patients with treatment-resistant epilepsy.

Conversion disorder or "psychogenic" syncope is a diagnosis of exclusion. It is more likely to occur in adolescents and under the following conditions: (1) when there is an audience, (2) when the episodes are long, (3) in patients with a lack of hemodynamic or autonomic changes, and (4) when there is no associated injury. Patients are typically calm when describing the episodes.

Important Elements in the History and Physical Examination (Figure 1)

History

Common benign

Neurocardiogenic syncope is usually provoked by prolonged standing, rising quickly from lying or sitting position, emotional circumstances, pain, or vigorous exercise in warm conditions. Presyncopal symptoms frequently occur before the syncopal episode and typically include light-headedness, dizziness, visual changes, headache, nausea, and diaphoresis. Injury is usually not significant since the prodrome alerts the patient to the impending syncope. Loss of consciousness is brief and patients quickly return to the normal state of alertness. There may be a brief episode of tonic-clonic activity but there is no postictal period. Bladder and bowel incontinence are not common findings, and do not help distinguish

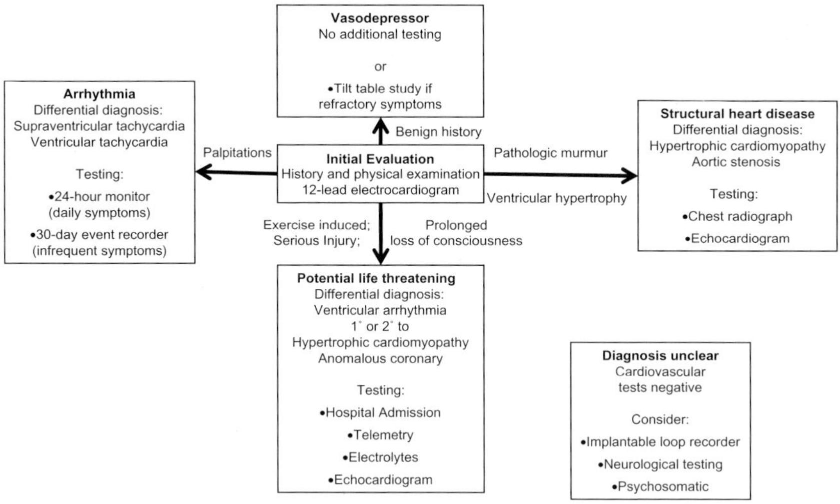

Figure 1. Diagnostic algorithm for evaluation of syncope.

neurocardiogenic syncope from a seizure. Family history is usually positive, other members experience similar benign fainting episodes.

Pathological findings

(1) *Exercise-related* syncope is concerning when it occurs during peak exercise. However, syncope is not uncommon immediately after exercise or with brief pauses in activity, and may be related to hemodynamic changes. Athletes who are able to assist in their own recovery are unlikely to have life-threatening arrhythmia.

(2) *Sudden loss of consciousness* and *serious injury* are concerning for ventricular arrhythmias. In contrast, patients with supraventricular tachycardia may experience preceding palpitations, dyspnea, and lightheadedness.

(3) *Congestive heart failure* may be suggested by cardiovascular symptoms of excessive fatigue, dyspnea with exertion or at rest, and diaphoresis. A history of recent viral illness should raise a suspicion for possible myocarditis. Diagnostic studies should include a 12-lead electrocardiogram and a chest radiograph to evaluate for cardiomegaly.

(4) *Family history* of sudden death should be examined carefully. In most cases, underlying risk factors can be found, including a history of coronary artery disease or chronic heart failure. However, deaths in multiple family members should be evaluated further for possible inherited conditions and structural cardiac abnormalities. Unexplained cases of seizures or drowning should be evaluated for potential long QT syndrome.

Physical examination

A complete physical examination should be performed in all pediatric patients with syncope including vital signs and orthostatic measurements.

(1) *Orthostatic hypotension* is defined by a 20 mm Hg decrease in systolic blood pressure and/or a decrease in diastolic blood pressure of at least 10 mm Hg within 3 minutes of standing. There is usually an associated increase in the heart rate of 15 to 20 beats per minute. Multiple techniques are used to obtain orthostatic hemodynamic analysis. One option includes measuring blood pressure and heart rate after 3–5 minutes in the lying, sitting, and standing positions. The patient should be monitored closely for any associated symptoms that may be more helpful than a change in vital signs.

(2) *Cardiac examination* should include visualization and palpation of the precordium to evaluate for cardiac chamber enlargement, as well as auscultation for accessory heart sounds.

(a) *Aortic stenosis* is represented by a systolic ejection murmur with an ejection click at the right upper sternal border. Peripheral pulses should be palpated thoroughly due to the increased risk of coarctation of the aorta.
(b) *Hypertrophic obstructive cardiomyopathy* is represented by a systolic ejection murmur along the left sternal border; one that increases in intensity when arising from a squatting position or with Valsalva maneuver. All adolescents should undergo cardiac auscultation with squatting-to-standing maneuvers during routine examinations.
(c) *Diastolic murmurs* are suspicious for pathology and require further evaluation, even if syncope or other symptoms are not present.
(d) An *S3 or S4 gallop*, elevated jugular venous pressure, rales, and hepatomegaly are suggestive of congestive heart failure and should prompt further evaluation.

(3) *An age-appropriate neurological examination* should be performed on all patients with syncope. Focal abnormalities may warrant further investigation or subspecialty referral.

Diagnostic tests

Routine

(1) *12-lead electrocardiogram* should be obtained at baseline to rule out cardiac causes of syncope. A review of standard interval and voltage measurements is

outside the scope of this chapter, but age-appropriate normal findings should be verified by reference. Abnormal findings which require further evaluation include:

(a) Left or right ventricular hypertrophy.
(b) Complete atrioventricular heart block.
(c) Mobitz Type II second-degree atrioventricular block. In contrast, Mobitz Type I (Wenckebach) second-degree atrioventricular block is common in many adolescents.
(d) Prolonged QT using the longest interval and correcting for heart rate (Bazett's formula: $QT/\sqrt{RR}$). In general, any corrected QT interval greater than 0.45 seconds should be considered abnormal, with worsening prognosis if 0.50 seconds or greater.
(e) Wolff-Parkinson-White syndrome characterized by shortened PR interval (< 0.11 seconds or age appropriate) and delta-wave.
(f) Brugada pattern characterized by an incomplete right bundle branch block with ST elevation in the anterior precordial leads.
(g) Arrhythmogenic right ventricular cardiomyopathy characterized by an epsilon wave, or terminal notching in the QRS complex.

Advanced

(1) *Echocardiography* is generally not helpful and need not be included in the routine work-up of syncope. However, directed evaluation may be indicated in verifying findings suggestive of ventricular hypertrophy or significant outflow tract obstruction.

(2) *Ambulatory holter and event monitoring* may be used to evaluate symptoms suggestive of arrhythmia (e.g. palpitations), but their diagnostic value is often limited. Twenty-four–hour monitors are rarely useful unless symptoms occur daily. A 30-day event monitor is more appropriate when symptoms are sporadic and unpredictable, although the odds of capturing an event may be very small. The presence or absence of asymptomatic ventricular ectopy has very low specificity. However, if ventricular arrhythmia is likely to be the cause of syncope, the patient should be admitted to a monitored bed until lethal tachyarrhythmias have been ruled out or treated.

(3) *Head-up tilt table testing* varies by protocol among laboratories, but usually involves inclining patients to a passive tilt angle of 60 to 80 degrees for a period of 15 to 45 minutes. Some centers also restrict fluids and recline patients prior to testing. In susceptible patients, a decrease in venous return is not fully compensated. Increased sympathetic tone results in recruitment of cardiac C fibers which

stimulate the medullary vasodepressor region. There is an abrupt withdrawal of sympathetic tone and increase in vagal tone, resulting in vasodilatation and syncope. Given that the goal is to reproduce the patient's symptoms, isoproterenol or nitroglycerin may be needed to elicit syncope.

Indications for testing include unexplained recurrent syncope, or an episode associated with injury in the absence of other organic causes. Tilt study is only positive in 30% to 75% of patients with syncope of unknown etiology. In addition, the reproducibility has not been demonstrated, and serial testing to evaluate pharmacologic treatments is of limited value. Children may be more susceptible than adults to orthostatic stress, and pre-syncope symptoms or frank syncope may be elicited in over half of normal control subjects. Sensitivity and specificity are also altered by patient co-operation, and findings may be questionable in young children who are easily distracted and cannot remain passively inclined for the duration of testing.

(4) *Electrophysiology testing's* yield is highest in patients with ischemic cardiomyopathy, depressed left ventricular ejection fraction, and non-sustained ventricular tachycardia. A signal averaged electrocardiogram may be helpful predicting whether a patient will have a diagnostic electrophysiology study. The technique is of limited value for patients with non-ischemic cardiomyopathy, and not commonly indicated in the pediatric population.

(5) *Implantable loop recorders* are newer monitoring devices which can record electrocardiographic data automatically, or be activated by a patient after a syncopal event. The technique may be useful in identifying symptomatic sinus nodal dysfunction or tachyarrhythmia. Given the need for surgical implantation and high financial cost, the greatest diagnostic yield is in patients with recurrent syncope with uncertain diagnoses.

(6) *Neurological testing* is not generally helpful in the routine evaluation of patients with syncope. Brain magnetic resonance imaging, computed tomography, or electroencephalography are only indicated if the history or physical examination suggests a neurological lesion or seizure.

Treatment

Routine

General measures include aggressive fluid intake and instruction on abortive maneuvers. The majority of pediatric patients will respond to a significant increase in fluid intake. Adolescent patients should consume at least 64 ounces (1920 ml) of water daily, and more when they are active. Avoiding caffeinated beverages, and lightly salting foods may also provide benefit. Generally, patients are drinking enough when their urine is colorless and they are not thirsty.

To prevent syncope, recognition of the prodromal symptoms is essential. At the onset of symptoms, patients should position themselves in the supine position with legs raised. Additional helpful maneuvers include crossing legs, standing on toes and tensing leg muscles, or performing isometric arm exercises. These maneuvers are designed to improve systemic venous return to the heart and avert a syncopal episode.

Advanced

Medications

(1) *Fludrocortisone* is a potent mineralocorticoid with minimal glucocorticoid activity. It promotes increased reabsorption of sodium and loss of potassium from the distal tubules in the kidney. The increased absorption of sodium leads to increased intravascular volume that may ameliorate symptoms. The usual dose in children and adolescents is 0.05–0.1 mg/day; the medication is usually well tolerated. Adverse effects may occur when using high doses. They include hypertension, hypokalemia, edema, headaches, and acne.

(2) *Beta-blockers* as a drug class may have multiple effects in treating neurocardiogenic syncope, including preventing stimulation and activation of the left ventricular mechanoreceptors which are responsible for the withdrawal of sympathetic tone, as well as blunting adrenergically mediated arterial vasodilation. Patients who require isoproterenol to provoke syncope are more likely to respond to beta-blocker therapy. Potential side effects include bradycardia, hypotension, fatigue, nausea, and diarrhea.

(3) *Alpha-adrenergic agonists* induce venous- and arterial-vasoconstriction through stimulation of α-sympathetic receptors of the peripheral vascular smooth muscle. Therefore, they enhance ventricular preload and prevent stimulation of ventricular mechoreceptors associated with low volume. Midodrine hydrochloride has been used successfully, although there are no clinical trials in the pediatric population. Benefits may be outweighed by side effects including: paresthesia, urinary urgency or retention, dysuria and polyuria, piloerection, and pruritus.

(4) *Selective serotonin-reuptake inhibitors* may have a role in attenuating the sympathetic nervous system's effects; although the exact mechanism for this action is not well understood. These agents may be useful in syncope associated with strong emotional stimuli including: visualization of blood, or physical pain. Side effects include sleep disturbance, anxiety, irritability, and suicidal

ideation in children and adolescents who are being treated for major depressive disorder.

Cardiac pacing

Permanent dual-chamber pacing may be used for patients with syncope refractory to other therapies. It should be reserved for the most difficult to manage cases. The results of unblinded randomized trials suggested a potential benefit in preventing syncope, although a subsequent single blinded trial failed to show a significant reduction in time to first recurrence. That said, cardiac pacing may still have a role in the management of syncope, especially in patients with insufficient prodrome, profound bradycardia, or asystole-associated syncope.

Driving Recommendations

Restrictions are governed by state law, and may be indicated in some patients with recurrent syncope.

Referral to Cardiovascular Medicine

Syncope is a common diagnosis of referral to pediatric and adult cardiology. In cases of probable benign vasodepressor syncope, the general practitioner may consider empirical management via patient education with emphasis on adequate fluid intake and abortive maneuvers. Patients with refractory symptoms may benefit from cardiology consultation for additional drug therapy. If there is a strong suspicion of structural abnormality or arrhythmia, referral to cardiology for further evaluation and testing is indicated. Patients with concerning presentation, including serious injury or strongly suspected ventricular arrhythmia, should be admitted for telemetry monitoring and in-depth evaluation.

References

Batra AS, Balaji S. Management of syncope in pediatric patients. *Curr Treat Options Cardiovasc Med.* 2005.7:391–398.

Driscoll DJ, Jacobsen SJ, Porter CJ, *et al.* Syncope in children and adolescents. *J Am Coll Cardiol.* 1997.29:1039–1045.

Grubb BP. Neurocardiogenic Syncope. *N Engl J Med.* 2005.352:1004–1010.

Strickberger SA, Benson DW, Biaggioni I, *et al.* AHA/ACCF Scientific statement on the evaluation of syncope. *J Am Coll Cardiol.* 2006.47:473–384.

18

CENTRAL NERVOUS SYSTEM INFECTIONS IN NEONATES, INFANTS, AND CHILDREN

Rebecca Wallihan and Dennis Cunningham

Introduction

Meningitis is defined as inflammation of the meninges, the linings covering the brain and spinal cord, and can be caused by bacterial, viral, and fungal pathogens. The condition can also be non-infectious in nature. Meningitis is often divided into two broad categories: septic and aseptic (bacterial and non-bacterial is a more appropriate classification). These categories, however, are not absolute. Some bacteria, especially atypical bacteria, can cause an illness more consistent with non-bacterial meningitis. For the purposes of this chapter, we apply the term bacterial meningitis to the illness caused by pyogenic bacteria. The term aseptic meningitis is used to describe meningitis caused by viruses, atypical bacteria, and fungi. Encephalitis refers to inflammation of the brain, while meningoencephalitis indicates inflammation of both the brain and meninges.

Bacterial Meningitis

Etiology

Bacterial meningitis is more common in the first month of life than at any other time. In the neonatal period, *Streptococcus agalactiae* (Group B *Streptococcus*),

---

Division of Infectious Diseases, Nationwide Children's Hospital and The Ohio State University, Columbus, Ohio, USA

Table 1. Causes of bacterial meningitis.

Age group	Pathogens
< 1 month	*S. agalactiae* *E. coli* Other enteric Gram negative bacilli (*Klebsiella* spp., *Enterobacter* spp., *Citrobacter* spp., etc.) *L. monocytogenes* *S. pneumoniae* *S. pyogenes* *H. influenzae*
1–3 months	*S. agalactiae* Gram negative bacilli (see neonatal pathogens) *S. pneumoniae* *N. meningitidis* *H. influenzae*
> 3 months	*S. pneumoniae* *N. meningitidis* *H. influenzae*

Escherichia coli, other enteric Gram negative bacilli, and *Listeria monocytogenes* are the most common bacterial pathogens. Less commonly, *Streptococcus pneumoniae*, *Streptococcus pyogenes* (Group A *Streptococcus*), and *Haemophilus influenzae* can be causative agents in this age group. In the 1–3-month age group, *S. agalactiae* is still the most common cause. Other meningitis pathogens in this age group include *S. pneumoniae* and *Neisseria meningitidis.* After 3 months of age, *S. pneumoniae* and *N. meningitidis* are seen most frequently, although *H. influenzae* can also be seen, especially in children who have not received the *H. influenzae B* vaccine. See Table 1 for common causes of bacterial meningitis according to age group.

Clinical features

The clinical features of bacterial meningitis vary according to age. The classic triad of fever, nuchal rigidity, and altered mental status is not commonly seen in neonates and infants; and the complete triad is present in less than half of children with meningitis. In neonates, meningitis may present with nonspecific symptoms and be clinically indistinguishable from sepsis. Patients in this age group can present with a wide variety of symptoms including fever or hypothermia, irritability, lethargy, feeding difficulty, emesis, or respiratory difficulty. Older infants and children with bacterial meningitis can also have a variable presentation, but will typically have fever or hypothermia plus neurological signs (e.g. irritability, headache, photophobia, or altered mental status). Seizures are common and can be the presenting feature in up to half of neonates and one third of children with bacterial meningitis.

Physical examination is often non-focal in neonates and young infants, but may reveal evidence of nuchal rigidity and increased intracranial pressure (ICP) [e.g. bulging fontanelle, cranial nerve palsies, or papilledema (rare)]. Kernig and Brudzinski signs may be found in older children, but their absence does not rule out meningitis. Kernig sign is when laying supine, with hips and knees flexed at 90°, the patient cannot extend the knee more than 135° or there is flexion of the opposite knee. Brudzinski sign is when laying supine, passive flexion of the neck causes back pain and the patient will flex their knees to relieve the discomfort.

Diagnosis

When meningitis is suspected, it is imperative to perform a lumbar puncture (LP) to aid in the diagnosis. The case history and the patient's physical examination may suggest meningitis but the definitive diagnosis is made through laboratory examination of the cerebrospinal fluid (CSF). Ideally, CSF should be obtained prior to administering antibiotics. This is often not feasible for unstable patients or those in whom radiological evaluation is necessary prior to performing an LP. Although initiating antibiotic treatment may cause the Gram stain or bacterial culture to be negative, there will still be abnormalities in protein and glucose content as well as in the cell count, to suggest meningitis. Overlap in CSF parameters can be seen with bacterial, viral, fungal, and tuberculous meningitis. In Table 2, we provide general guidelines for interpreting CSF studies.

The definitive diagnosis of bacterial meningitis relies on isolation of a bacterial pathogen from the CSF. A presumptive diagnosis of bacterial meningitis is made in patients with a positive bacterial blood culture and CSF pleocytosis, even with a negative CSF bacterial culture. Bacterial blood cultures may, however, be negative in up to one third of neonates and one half of children with bacterial meningitis. In cases with negative bacterial cultures, or when aseptic meningitis is suspected, additional laboratory testing may be necessary. Viral cultures may be helpful when viral meningitis is suspected, but the result of this test may take a few days. Alternatively, many viruses and some bacteria can be detected using polymerase chain reaction (PCR) assays. Although the authors of several studies have suggested that serum inflammatory markers, such as procalcitonin and C-reactive protein, may be helpful in differentiating viral and bacterial meningitis, there is not enough data to recommend their routine use when making clinical decisions.

Table 2. CSF in meningitis.

	Opening pressure (mm H_2O)	Leukocytes (cells/mm^3)	%PMNs‡	Protein (mg/dl)	Glucose (mg/dl)
Normal (beyond neonatal period)	50–80	<5	0	20–45 (up to 100 in < 1 month of age)	>50% simultaneous blood sugar (75% in neonates)
Viral	100–150	<500*	20–40%	Nl or <100	Nl or slightly decreased
Bacterial	100–300	>1000	>85–90%	>100–150	Undetectable to <40%
Fungal	180–300	<500	<10–20%	>100–200	<40%
Tuberculous	180–300	<300	<10–20%	>200–300	<40%
Brain abscess	100–300	<500	20–40%	Nl-slightly increased	Nl-slightly decreased

‡Polymorphonuclear white blood cells. *Enteroviruses can be associated with up to 3000 WBC and early in the course have a predominance of PMNs. Nl: normal limits.

Antimicrobial therapy

Empiric treatment of meningitis is based on the epidemiology of the most common pathogens for each age group. In Table 3, we list empiric therapy for suspected meningitis with a negative Gram stain.

If interpretation of the Gram stain suggests a specific etiology, the therapy is tailored to eradicate that pathogen. Use of broad spectrum antibiotics, however, should continue until the results of the bacterial culture and antibiotic susceptibilities become available. Table 4 lists the recommended empiric treatment based on a positive Gram stain.

Adjunctive therapies and supportive care

The use of dexamethasone has been shown to be beneficial in randomized controlled trials of meningitis in adults, but the use of steroids for children with suspected meningitis is still debated. The authors of several studies have shown that dexamethasone is effective in preventing hearing loss in *Haemophilus* meningitis. At this time, there is insufficient data to routinely use corticosteroids in bacterial meningitis due to other organisms; although, there may be some benefit

Table 3. Empiric therapy for suspected bacterial meningitis with negative Gram stain.

Age	Antibiotic therapy
< 1 month	Ampicillin **PLUS** Gentamicin **OR** Cefotaxime
1–3 months	Vancomycin* **PLUS** Ceftriaxone **OR** Cefotaxime
> 3 months	Vancomycin **PLUS** Ceftriaxone **OR** Cefotaxime

*Some experts recommend ampicillin in place of vancomycin in this age group unless the gram stain suggests *S. pneumoniae.*

Table 4. Antibiotic therapy by Gram stain and pathogen.

Gram stain	Likely pathogen	Recommended antibiotic therapy
Gram-positive diplococci	*S. pneumoniae*	Vancomycin **PLUS** Ceftriaxone **OR** Cefotaxime
Gram-negative diplococci	*N. meningitidis*	Ceftriaxone **OR** Cefotaxime
Pleomorphic gram-negative coccobacili	*H. influenzae*	Ceftriaxone **OR** Cefotaxime
Gram-positive rods and/or coccobacilli	*L. monocytogenes*	Ampicillin **PLUS** Gentamicin
Gram-positive cocci in chains	*S. agalactiae*	Ampicillin **PLUS** Gentamicin
Gram-negative bacilli	Enteric Gram-negative bacteria (e.g. *E. coli, Klebsiella* spp., etc.)	Ceftriaxone **OR** Cefotaxime **PLUS** Gentamicin (or other aminoglycoside)

in Pneumococcal meningitis. Therefore, most authorities currently recommend adjunctive treatment with dexamethasone 0.15 mg/kg/dose every 6 hours prior to or concomitant with the first dose of antibiotics in children older than 6 weeks of age with suspected *Haemophilus* or Pneumococcal meningitis (after carefully weighing the risks and benefits).

Patients with suspected meningitis must be monitored closely for evidence of increased ICP. This includes frequent vital signs and neurological assessment. At least daily measurement of head circumference is recommended in infants and children less than 18 months of age.

Although fluid restriction was previously considered standard of care for patients with bacterial meningitis, more recently it has fallen out of favor. Parenteral hydration should be used to keep the mean arterial blood pressure $> 95^{th}$ percentile. This allows the cerebral perfusion pressure to be maintained despite elevation in ICP. Fluid restriction is only advised in adequately hydrated patients with evidence of syndrome of inappropriate antidiuretic hormone secretion (e.g. hyponatremia).

Complications

When pooling data from all age groups, the mortality from bacterial meningitis is less than 10%. This figure, however, is higher in neonates and in patients with Pneumococcal meningitis. As mentioned previously, seizures are not uncommon in patients with bacterial meningitis. Specifically, seizures tend to be more common early in the course of the illness. When seizures occur after the acute phase, they are usually associated with neurological sequelae. Subdural effusions are seen in up to one third of patients with bacterial meningitis, and are more commonly seen with *H. influenzae* and Pneumococcal disease. Subdural effusions tend to resolve spontaneously. Subdural empyema, defined as a collection of pus between the duramater and arachnoid layers, is a less frequent complication seen in approximately 2% of patients with meningitis. While subdural effusions generally resolve spontaneously, empyemas require surgical drainage. Intracranial abscess is a well-described complication of bacterial meningitis, especially in neonates. It is most commonly seen in newborns with meningitis caused by *Citrobacter*, *Enterobacter*, or *Proteus spp.*

The most common long term complication of bacterial meningitis in children is hearing loss; it is more frequently seen when the pathogen is *Pneumococcus*. Other potential sequelae include cognitive impairment, behavioral problems, developmental delay (including speech and motor impairment), decreased visual acuity, and seizures.

Table 5. Causes of aseptic meningitis.

Common	Uncommon	
• Enteroviruses • Herpes simplex virus • Arboviruses (eastern equine encephalitis, western equine encephalitis, St. Louis encephalitis, California encephalitis, West Nile) • *Borrelia burgdorferi* (Lyme disease)	• Respiratory viruses (Influenza, parainfluenza, adenovirus, human metapneumovirus) • Other herpesviruses (Epstein-Barr virus, varicella-zoster virus, cytomegalovirus, human herpesvirus 6) • Rabies • Human immunodeficiency virus • Mumps • Measles	• Lymphocytic choriomeningitis virus • Rotavirus • Parvovirus B19 • *Rickettsia rickettsii* • *Mycoplasma pneumoniae* • *Mycobacterium tuberculosis* • *Bartonella henselae* • Fungi (*Cryptococcus, Coccidioides, Histoplasma, Blastomyces, Candida*) • Parasites (*Taenia solium, Toxoplasma gondii*)

Aseptic Meningitis, Encephalitis, and Meningoencephalitis

Etiology

When considering causes of aseptic meningitis in infants and children, Enteroviruses are by far the most commonly seen pathogens. These organisms account for up to 95% of cases. Members of the Herpesviridae family can also cause meningitis, with herpes simplex viruses being the most common and arguably the most important because of the potential for severe disease and complications. While the Arboviruses typically cause encephalitis, they can also cause meningitis or meningoencephalitis. Some bacterial causes of aseptic meningitis include *Borrelia burgdorferi, Rickettsia rickettsii*, and *Mycoplasma pneumoniae.* Meningitis can also be caused by pathogens other than viruses and bacteria, including fungi and parasites, but these infections are primarily seen in immunocompromised hosts and will only be mentioned briefly. In Table 5, we list some of the common and uncommon pathogens which cause aseptic meningitis.

Clinical features

The presentation of aseptic meningitis can be similar to that of bacterial meningitis, although the symptoms tend to be less severe, especially in older infants and children. The exception to this statement is infection with herpes simplex virus types I and II. In neonates, the infection can present as a serious case of shock and purpura fulminans. In addition to the common signs and symptoms of meningitis, the presentation may suggest specific viruses, such as rash, conjunctivitis, pharyngitis or herpangina.

Diagnosis

In cases with negative blood and CSF cultures, or when aseptic meningitis is suspected, additional laboratory testing may be needed. Viral culture may be helpful when viral meningitis is suspected, but the results may not become available in a timely manner. Identification of enterovirus may require 2 or 3 weeks. HSV is notoriously difficult to grow in CSF culture (5% sensitivity). If HSV is on the differential, the CSF should be evaluated using PCR for HSV.

Treatment

Corticosteroids are not routinely recommended in the management of patients with aseptic meningitis, except for those with tuberculous meningitis. In the United States, this has become an unusual condition. Thus, consultation with an infectious diseases expert is advised.

HSV

Treatment of patients with IV acyclovir is considered standard of care. In children < 6 months of age, the dose is 20 mg/kg IV q8 hours. For older children and adults, the dose is 10 mg/kg IV every 8 hours. Because acyclovir is a well tolerated medication, some experts use 20 mg/kg IV every 8 hours regardless of the child's age. Of note, oral acyclovir is not adequate treatment for HSV encephalitis.

Enterovirus

Enterovirus encephalitis generally has an excellent prognosis for full recovery. Seizures are relatively rare in children with Enterovirus encephalitis. Care is supportive. There are no antiviral agents to treat Enterovirus. In patients with hypogammaglobulinema, IVIG therapy may be useful.

References

Chávez-Bueno S, McCracken GHJ. Bacterial meningitis in children. *Pediatr Clin North Am.* 2005.52:795–810.

Cherry JD. Recognition and management of encephalitis in children. *Adv Exp Med Biol.* 2009.634:53–60.

Kim KS. Acute bacterial meningitis in infants and children. *Lancet Infect Dis.* 2010.1:32.

Long SS, Pickering LK, Prober CG (eds.). *Principles and Practice of Pediatric Infectious Diseases.* 3rd ed. Philadelphia: Saunders. 2009.

Tunkel AR, Glaser CA, Bloch KC, *et al.* Infectious diseases society of america. the management of encephalitis: clinical practice guidelines by the Infectious Diseases society of america. *Clin Infect Dis.* 2008.47(3):303–327.

Tunkel AR, Hartman BJ, Kaplan SL, *et al.* Practice guidelines for the management of bacterial meningitis. *Clin Infect Dis.* 2004.39(9):1267–1284.

19

HYDROCEPHALUS

Eric M. Jackson and Corey Raffel†*

An 11-month-old boy was brought to the neurosurgery clinic for evaluation of hydrocephalus. According to his parents, the boy was noted to have a "large head" most of his life, but the growth has yet to level off. The boy has exhibited episodes of head turning which were concerning for seizures, so the child's pediatrician ordered a CT scan of the head. The images revealed enlargement of the boy's lateral and third ventricles, with a normal-size forth ventricle. The radiologist's assessment was that the child had aqueductal stenosis. An MRI of the brain was performed; interpretation of the test confirmed the diagnosis of aqueductal stenosis (Figure 1).

On physical examination, the child was awake, alert and interactive. His pupils were equal, round and reactive to light. He was able to track objects of his interest in all directions. The boy had a small anterior fontanelle that was flat. The head circumference was measured at 51 cm, which was well above the 95th percentile for the child's age. After an extended conversation about treatment options, the child's parents elected to proceed with endoscopic third ventriculostomy (ETV). The boy underwent the procedure and was discharged the following evening in good condition. The boy was brought back to the neurosurgery clinic 2 weeks later for a follow-up visit. The child's mother indicated the boy was, overall, doing well. That said, it was the mother's assessment that the child was somewhat irritable and he did not like to lay down flat on his back. On physical examination, the child had a soft bulge at the side of the burr-hole used

*Division of Neurosurgery, Nationwide Children's Hospital and The Ohio State University, Columbus, Ohio, USA
†The Ohio State University, Columbus, Ohio, USA

for the ETV procedure. The boy's head circumference was measured at 52.5 cm. Based on the clinical findings, a limited MRI of the brain was performed. The test was interpreted as having evidence of re-enlargement of the ventricular system. Such finding was concerning for failure of the ETV. The surgeon discussed treatment options with the boy's parents. These included surgical reassessment of the ETV, or placing a ventriculo-peritoneal (VP) shunt. At the time of surgery, the third ventriculostomy was found to be widely patent (see Figure 2). These findings were suggestive of a CSF absorption problem. Thus, a VP shunt was placed. Following the procedure, the child's head circumference resumed normal growth.

Epidemiology

Surgical techniques to treat hydrocephalus with valve-regulated shunts are more than 50 years old. Despite the success of treatments for hydrocephalus, these conditions remain a major public health concern, and result in high cost to the health care system. At this time, about 300,000 people in the United States have

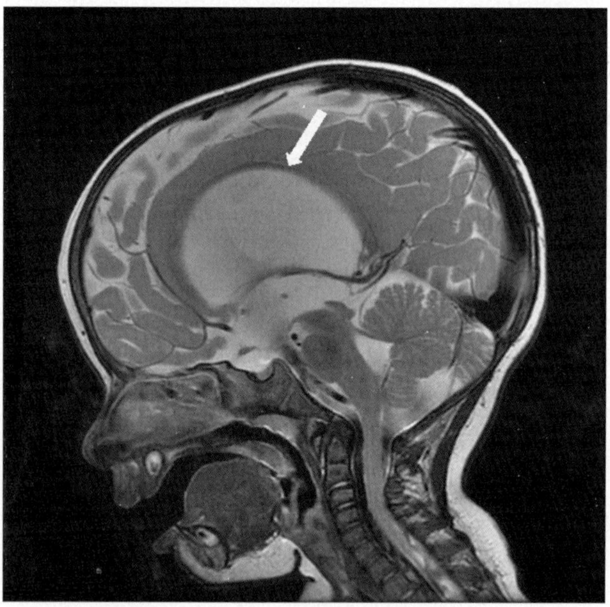

Figure 1. Sagital T2 weighted MRI of a patient with aqueductal stenosis and hydrocephalus. Arrow points at an enlarged lateral ventricle.

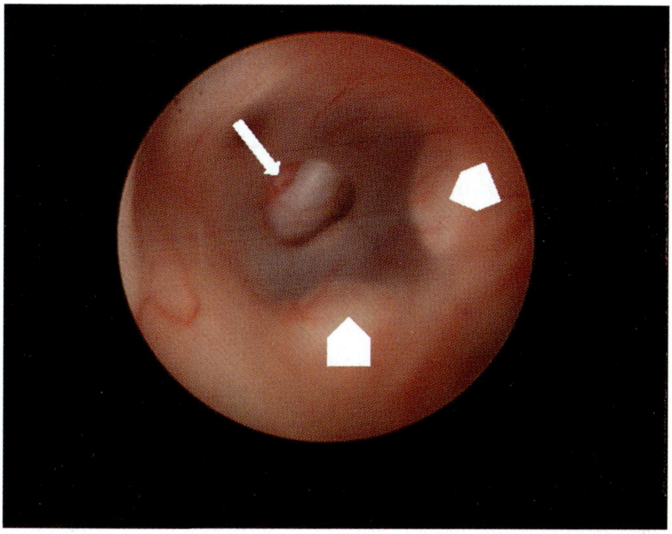

Figure 2. Endoscopic image of a patent opening in the floor of the third ventricle (arrow). The paired structures posterior to the opening (around 3 and 5 o'clock due to rotation) are the mammillary bodies (arrowheads).

hydrocephalus. The annual incidence of the condition is estimated at 11 per 100,000. These numbers suggest that hydrocephalus is more common than pediatric brain tumors, and as common as juvenile onset diabetes mellitus and cystic fibrosis. The cost of caring for patients with hydrocephalus in the United States is estimated to be 1 billion dollars annually. Clearly, hydrocephalus is a major public health problem. And primary care providers are bound to have patients with hydrocephalus in their practice.

Pathogenesis

At the most basic level, hydrocephalus occurs when the rate of CSF production in any compartment of the brain exceeds the rate of absorption. The location of the fluid collection and the associated signs and symptoms as well the treatment options depend on the underlying cause of the hydrocephalus and which ventricles are involved. The rate of CSF production, estimated to be 20 ml per hour or 480 ml per day, is quite constant and probably does not change much after 1 year of age. Under normal circumstances, the absorptive capacity exceeds the rate of production. With this in mind, there are two mechanism by which hydrocephalus develops. On one hand, there may be impaired CSF egress from the ventricular system to the site of absorption, i.e. the arachnoid granulations. On the other hand, obstruction at the level of the arachnoid granulations reduces their CSF-absorptive capacity. The first type described is called non-communicating or obstructive hydrocephalus, and the second one is called communicating hydrocephalus.

Blockage to CSF flow most often occurs at the aqueduct of Sylvius. This small channel, measuring approximately 2 mm in diameter, connects the third ventricle with the fourth ventricle. Blockage at the aqueduct is the most common cause of congenital hydrocephalus. Aqueductal stenosis can also occur later in life; these patients are thought to have scarring or some other acquired process resulting in loss of patency of the channel. Stenosis of the aqueduct can usually be identified either by CT scan of the head or MRI of the brain. In those instances, the lateral and third ventricles are dilated, but the fourth ventricle, because its distal location to the blockage of CSF flow, is normal in size. This condition is sometimes referred to as "triventricular hydrocephalus." Brain MRI CSF-flow studies reveal the absence of fluid flow across the aqueduct.

Although uncommon, hydrocephalus may occur from abnormalities at the foramina of Munro. These foramina are the passageway for CSF between the two lateral ventricles and third ventricle. If one foramen is occluded, only one lateral ventricle will be enlarged. This may occur through formation of a membrane or scaring. If both foramina are occluded, e.g. a tumor growing in the area, both lateral ventricles will be dilated.

Occasionally, hydrocephalus is caused by occlusion of the outlets of the fourth ventricle. These are the paired lateral foramina of Luschka, and the midline foramen of Magendie. The most common cause of foramina occlusion is presence of a tumor in the cerebellum or the fourth ventricle, which are relatively common locations of tumors in children. In addition, obstruction of the outlets of the fourth ventricle can occur due to inflammation and scar formation. In premature infants, this situation most commonly occurs after intraventricular hemorrhage; especially when associated to CNS infection.

Hydrocephalus is also common in children born with open neural-tube defects, i.e. myelomeningocele. The exact nature of the hydrocephalus in these children is not clear, and it is most likely multifactorial. The small size of the posterior fossa with crowding of its contents and the associated Chiari type 2 malformation are likely causative factors.

Scars in the subarachnoid space may also lead to hydrocephalus. As CSF leaves the ventricular system, it must flow through the basal cisterns into the cortical subarachnoid space to get access to the site of CSF absorption at the arachnoid granulations. Diseases that cause scarring of the subarachnoid space in the basal cisterns, over the surface of the brain and at the arachnoid granulations include: hemorrhage, trauma, premature birth, and meningitis. Tuberculous meningitis has a predilection for the basal cisterns. Thus, hydrocephalus may be the initial presentation of this condition.

Signs and Symptoms

With the routine use of the fetal sonography, the diagnosis of hydrocephalus can potentially be made prenatally. When the diagnosis is made during the first trimester, the hydrocephalus is often a consequence of severe derangement of brain development, and the prognosis for reasonable neurological outcome is grim. When the diagnosis is made later in gestation, the outcome is more difficult to predict. In the later situation, 30% of patients will develop progressive hydrocephalus (ventricles which continue to increase in size); 30% of patients will have evidence of stable ventriculomegaly (the ventricles remain the same size); and in 30% of patients the ventricle size will decrease (resolving hydrocephalus). In the last case, the most important variable is the coexistence of other congenital anomalies. If present, they significantly worsen the prognosis. Because the course of *in utero* hydrocephalus detected late in pregnancy is so variable, treatment is delayed until the child is born. The signs and symptoms of postnatal hydrocephalus depend on the child's age at the time of diagnosis. Because cranial sutures are not closed in infants, the head can expand and accommodate a large volume of CSF. Thus, in this age group, abnormally rapid head growth is a more common presentation of hydrocephalus than symptoms of raised intracranial pressure. These children will have a bulging anterior fontanelle and diastasis of the cranial sutures. The "classic" presentation of neonatal hydrocephalus, with bulging anterior fontanelle, prominent scalp veins, and forced downward gaze (sunset sign) may occur — but like most other classic presentations, it is uncommon.

Beyond infancy, the signs and symptoms of hydrocephalus are those of raised intracranial pressure. These include: headache, emesis, and lethargy. Headaches are especially concerning when they become progressively worse over time, or when associated with lethargy, behavior changes, and diplopia. Headaches from raised intracranial pressure may wake the child up from sleep or be present upon waking up in the morning. Emesis is associated with headaches that occur in the morning, and the child may experience temporary relief of the headaches after the emesis. Papilledema is a salient feature of raised intracranial pressure and is usually present in children with hydrocephalus. The retina must be examined for signs of papilledema when raised intracranial pressure is suspected. An important caveat is that the signs and symptoms just described are also those of other conditions that may also cause raised intracranial pressure. Such conditions include idiopathic intracranial hypertension (pseudotumor cerebri) and brain tumors, either with or without associated hydrocephalus.

Diagnostic Studies

Magnetic resonance imaging is the study of choice when hydrocephalus is being considered. MRI scans provide the best anatomical detail and help identify the site of the CSF's flow block. MRI is an important tool to determine if endoscopic third ventriculostomy is a treatment option. The disadvantages to the use of MRI are high cost and the time required to obtain the images. Infants and young children will also need to be sedated or given general anesthesia. A solution is to screen children using a limited study. This consists of a single series of T2- weighted axial images. This option does not provide the anatomical detail of a full MRI scan but the information it provides helps identify hydrocephalus. Head CT may also be used to screen children for hydrocephalus. The study can be performed quickly, thus avoiding the need for sedation or general anesthesia. Also, CT scanners are more likely to be available than MRI scanners. The disadvantages to CT imaging include less anatomic details, and the delivery of a dose of radiation to the child's head. Other than availability, a CT scan has few advantages over the limited MRI study used for screening purposes as described above.

In infants with an open anterior fontanelle, cranial sonography can also be used as a screening tool for hydrocephalus. The study can be used to identify dilation of the ventricles, but does not provide the anatomical detail of either a CT scan of the head or an MRI of the brain. If hydrocephalus is identified by sonography, at least one MRI scan prior to any surgical treatment is necessary. In infants sonography is especially useful for the purpose of following the size of the ventricles after treatment. In addition, serial cranial sonograms can be used to follow the size of the ventricles of premature infants who have suffered an intraventricular hemorrhage.

Treatment of Hydrocephalus and its Complications

The use of shunts has revolutionized the treatment of, and outcomes for, children with hydrocephalus (Figure 3). A shunt consists of three parts: (1) a catheter placed into the lateral ventricle; (2) a valve to control flow through the shunt; and (3) a catheter extending from the valve to the eventual site of CSF absorption. The most common site for extracranial cerebrospinal fluid absorption is the peritoneal cavity; hence the name ventriculoperitoneal shunt (VP shunt). Alternative locations are used in circumstances when the peritoneal cavity does not absorb the fluid properly. Common alternative locations include: the right atrium of the heart (usually via

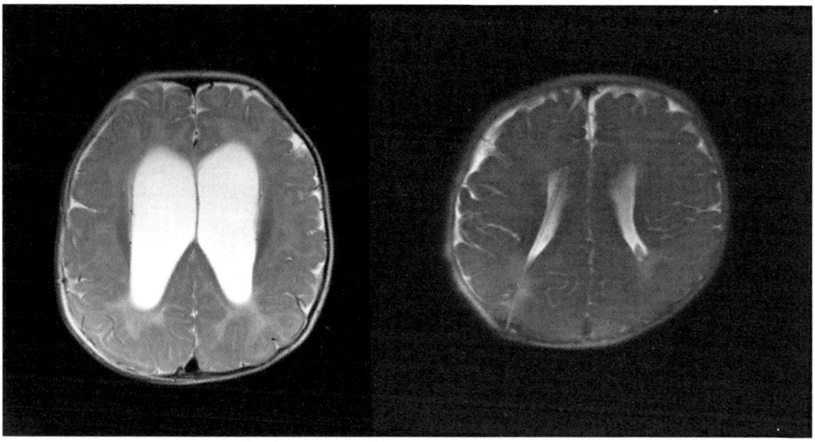

Figure 3. T2 axial images of a patient with hydrocephalus (a) pre- and (b) post-shunting.

the internal jugular vein or other large vein), the pleural cavity, the gallbladder, the urinary system, and the sagittal sinus.

A dizzying array of shunt hardware is available with various catheter designs, various valves which work on different engineering principles, programmable valves where the pressure required to open the valve can be adjusted, and antibiotic-impregnated hardware to decrease the incidence of infection. Disappointingly so, there is essentially no scientific evidence to suggest that one piece of hardware is better than the other. Thus, the hardware selection process is dictated almost exclusively by the surgeon's preferences.

VP shunts have the great advantage of successfully treating hydrocephalus immediately after placement. They have the disadvantages of failure or blockage, infection, and over-shunting. Shunts are simply plumbing, and like plumbing, they are prone to failure. Approximately 50% of shunts placed while the child is an infant fail within 2 years of implantation. Thus, patients with shunts require close follow-up. Patients with shunt failure present with the same signs and symptoms as those with hydrocephalus. As a caveat, however, papilledema is not always seen in patients with shunt failure. The most common presentation of shunt failure is that of a patient with emesis and headaches. Evidently, these symptoms are non-specific and commonly seen in patients with a viral illness. Nonetheless, a low index of suspicion for shunt failure must be maintained, because the consequences of missing a malfunctioning shunt can be serious. When a child presents with signs and symptoms of shunt failure, it is imperative that a radiological test be completed.

This will need to be compared to studies obtained when the patient was symptom-free. It is important to highlight that some patient's ventricles' may not change significantly with shunt malfunction. If the ventricles' size increases without any other apparent reason, shunt malfunction is the likely cause and surgical revision should be performed.

Because shunt placement involves implantation of foreign material, the risk of infection is higher than for most other neurosurgical procedures. The authors of a recent study reported that among 41 children's hospitals in the United States, shunt infection rate was anywhere between 2.5% and 12.3% per procedure. The incidence of shunt infection rises during the first few weeks that follow the procedure, and then falls to close to zero by 6 months. Infection is best treated by removal of the shunt hardware, placement of an external ventricular drain, and treatment of the infection with antibiotics. When the CSF cultures fail to grow pathogens, a new shunt can be implanted.

Over-shunting is a rare condition about which a great deal has been written. Radiographic findings in a patient at risk for developing over-shunting include ventricles that are small in size (slit ventricles) and thicker than normal skull bones (Figure 4). Patients with "slit ventricles syndrome" (SVS) may present with

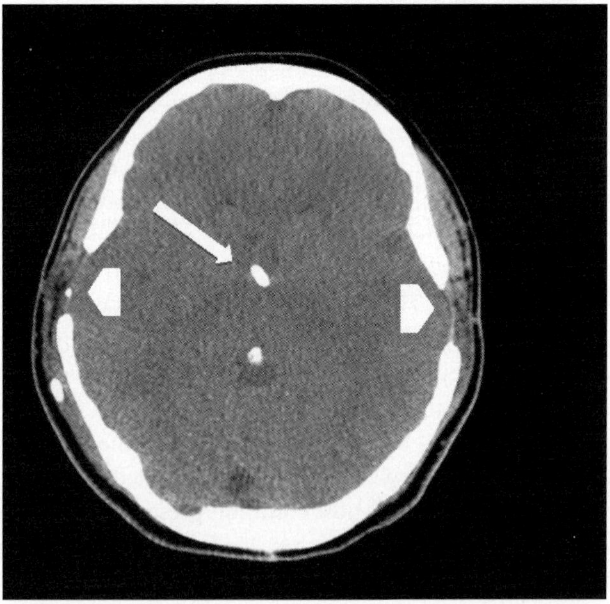

Figure 4. CT image of a patient with slit ventricles demonstrating the catheter in the 3rd ventricle (arrow). Of note, this patient had bilateral temporal decompressions as is evidenced by the bony defect bilaterally (arrowheads).

chronic headaches. That said, approximately 40% of adults who had shunts placed during childhood have frequent headaches. Some children with SVS experience intermittent signs of shunt failure that resolve without intervention. In such cases, the child may complain of severe headaches and may also be lethargic. Part of the paradox of SVS is that when a radiological test is completed in a patient, the ventricles' size appears to be at baseline. Some hypothesize that this syndrome is caused by intermittent occlusion of the ventricular catheter by the collapsing walls of a lateral ventricles. As pressure builds, the patient becomes symptomatic. Finally, the pressure rises to the point where it pushes the ventricle's wall away from the shunt. Given that there is no hardware malfunction or infection, the shunt starts working again, and the symptoms resolve. Over-shunting is a difficult condition to treat. Revisions of the shunt, the shunt valve, use of programmable valves, and the placement of an additional shunt have all been tried with varying success.

Because of the aforementioned complications, alternatives to VP shunts have been explored. Endoscopic third ventriculostomy is one of those alternatives. If hydrocephalus is a consequence of an obstruction at the aqueduct of Sylvius or the outlet of the fourth ventricle, surgical fenestration of the floor of the third ventricle will allow the CSF to escape the ventricular system via the extra-cerebral subarachnoid space. While the theory behind this procedure is sound, clinical practice has shown that fenestration is not always successful. Variables that suggest that the ETV will be unsuccessful include young age (less than 6 months), and instances where hydrocephalus is a consequence of a CNS infection. By carefully selecting patients based on age, cause of hydrocephalus, and whether the patient has had a previous shunt, the success rate can approach 90%. A prognostic ETV success score, one that takes these variables into consideration, has been developed. Like shunts, ETV may fail, but the overall failure rate is lower than that of shunts. The failure rate of ETV is high during the 6 months that follow the procedure. In the event of failure, either a repeat ETV or placement of a VP shunt is required.

References

Berry JG, Hall MA, Sharma V, *et al.* A multi-institutional, 5-year analysis of initial and multiple ventricular shunt revisions in children. *Neurosurgery.* 2008.62:445–454.

Drake JM, Kulkarni AV, Kestle J. Endoscopic third ventriculostomy versus ventriculoperitoneal shunt in pediatric patients: a decision analysis. *Childs Nerv Syst.* 2009.25: 467–472.

Kestle J, Drake J, Milner R, *et al.* Long-term follow-up data from the shunt design trial. *Pediatr Neurosurg.* 2000.33:230–236.

Kulkarni AV, Drake JM, Kestle JRW, *et al.* Endoscopic third ventriculostomy vs. cerebrospinal fluid shunt in the treatment of hydrocephalus in children: a propensity score-adjusted analysis. *Neurosurgery.* 2010.67:588–593.
Kulkarni AV, Drake JM, Mallucci CL, *et al.* Endoscopic third ventriculostomy in the treatment of childhood hydrocephalus. *J Pediatr.* 2009.155:254–259.
Simon TD, Hall M, Riva-Cambrin J, *et al.* Infection rates following initial cerebrospinal fluid shunt placement across pediatric hospitals. *J Neurosurg (Peds).* 2009.4:156–165.
Simon TD, Riva-Cambrin J, Srivastava R, *et al.* Hospital care for children with hydrocephalus in the United States: utilization, charges, comorbidities, and deaths. *J Neurosurg (Peds).* 2008.1:131–137.

20

NEUROLOGY OF THE NEONATE

Lenora Lehwald and Laurel Slaughter

A baby girl is born at full term to a 27-year-old mother. The child's birth is via emergency C-section because the mother presented to the hospital with severe vaginal bleeding, and placental abruption was suspected. The baby's Apgar scores are 0, 1, and 2 at 1, 5, and 10 minutes respectively. The baby's first arterial blood gas reveals a pH of 6.87 and a base deficit of −28. The baby is transported to a tertiary care hospital where she undergoes hypothermia protocol beginning at 3 hours of life. As per protocol, the child's EEG is continuously monitored. Initial interpretation of the EEG reveals suppressed background activity. Clinical seizures become evident soon thereafter. The seizures are controlled after multiple doses of phenobarbital and levetiracetam. The child is prescribed maintenance doses of these medications. When the hypothermia protocol is complete, MRI of the brain is performed. Interpretation of the test is compatible with severe hypoxic-ischemic injury involving cortical and subcortical areas as well as deep gray matter. Clinically, the child's muscle tone increases over the ensuing 3 days. The child remains encephalopathic through her hospital stay. Eventually, she is able to tolerate oral feeding, and is discharged home on maintenance anti-seizure medications.

Defining the Neonatal Population

A neonate, by definition, is an infant within the first 28 days of life. Most full-term neonates (> 37 weeks gestational age) are born without neurological problems.

Division of Child Neurology, Nationwide Children's Hospital and The Ohio State University, Columbus, Ohio, USA

Full-term infants, however, may experience a variety of neurological symptoms related to: hypoxic-ischemic injury, neonatal seizures, exposure to toxic substances, congenital or neonatal infections, congenital nervous system malformations, neonatal stroke or hemorrhage, and genetic or metabolic disorders. Premature infants can, of course, have the above. But in premature children, the more common concerns are those stemming from periventricular leukomalacia (white matter disease of prematurity) and intraventricular hemorrhage. The authors of a large cohort study reported that approximately 40% of very preterm infants (defined as < 33 weeks gestation) have long-term neurodevelopmental disabilities.

Clinical History of the Neonate

The clinical history of a neonate is different from that of other patient populations. The neonate's medical history is actually the history of the mother's pregnancy and the child's delivery. Pertinent information includes: the mother's age, obstetrical history, the results of laboratory and serological studies, history of prenatal medical care, presence of common pregnancy complications (hypertension, gestational diabetes, bleeding, and preterm labor), the date of last menses, infections, and exposure to toxic substances or those of abuse. The clinician should also gather information on labor and delivery such as type of delivery (if the child was delivered by a Cesarean section it is important to inquire the reason), duration of labor, presence of fever or bleeding, history of fetal distress, medications given to the mother (tocolytics, antibiotics, analgesics, corticosteroids, and sedating medications), meconium staining, and umbilical cord (henceforth "cord") or placental anomalies. It is also important to note the child's Apgar scores, initial cord-blood gases, and the other laboratory data.

The physical examination of a neonate is also distinctly different from that of an older child. While some limitations exist, much can be learned from careful observation, even before directly interacting with the baby. After unbundling the child, the clinician should evaluate the patient's level of alertness, quality and quantity of spontaneous movements, position of the child's limbs while at rest, spontaneous eye opening, and evidence of jitteriness or hypersensitivity to stimuli. The child's head shape and head circumference should be evaluated. It is important to look for signs of molding, swelling, and presence of fluid collections. The anterior fontanelle should be examined before the child becomes upset; it should be soft and flat. The remainder of the general examination is focused on looking for dysmorphic features, abnormal skin findings, asymmetry of limbs, spinal anomalies, and muscle contractures.

Neurological Examination of the Neonate in the Nursery or Neonatal Intensive Care Unit

The neurological examination begins by assessing the child's alertness, ease of arousal, and response to gentle noxious stimuli. The clinician should note the time of the exam relative to the baby's sleeping and feeding cycles; multiple examinations may be needed to get a true assessment of the baby's neurological status. The examination continues by testing the cranial nerves: pupillary reaction to light, the child's ability to fix on and follow an object or the examiner's face, extra ocular movements, corneal reflex, facial symmetry, attempts at sucking, and gag reflex. Next is the motor examination, often the most useful part of the neurological examination of a newborn. The child's posture at rest should be noted. The term infant tends to hold the arms and legs in gentle flexion at the knees and elbows (fetal position). Muscle strength, range of motion, and efforts at resisting the examination should be noted. Deep tendon reflexes can usually be elicited at the patellae, ankles, and biceps and pectoralis muscles. The plantar response may be difficult to interpret because of competing reflexes, but persistent asymmetries should be noted. The presence of 5–10 beats of clonus at the ankles may be normal in a neonate, unless it is persistently asymmetric. Sensory reaction to gentle touch, or if necessary noxious stimuli, should be noted. The final piece of the neurological assessment in the newborn is looking for developmental reflexes such as the Moro reflex, palmar and plantar grasps, and "fencing" (asymmetric tonic neck) reflex. Important to the interpretation of the above findings is the assessment of the gestational age using standardized tools such as the Ballard scoring system.

Common Neurological Diseases of the Neonate

Hypoxic-ischemic injury (neonatal encephalopathy)

Probably the most commonly encountered neurological problem in the neonatal period is hypoxic-ischemic encephalopathy (HIE). A cerebral insult due to poor perfusion or oxygenation may be prenatal (placental insufficiency or hemorrhage, inflammation, infection), during labor or delivery, during the resuscitation after delivery, or a combination of the above. Therefore, the mechanism is often referred to as perinatal (around the time of birth) asphyxia. In most cases, it is difficult to determine the exact timing of an injury, and multiple factors may be involved, therefore identifying a specific cause of the HIE, is often not possible. HIE, as the name implies, is caused by a combination of poor cerebral perfusion, and lack of oxygenation. At the cellular level, selective neuronal necrosis occurs within the first hours due to ATP depletion. This is followed by rapid reperfusion which also contributes to the injury. There is also ongoing secondary injury that occurs over the next hours to several days. The secondary cellular injury is thought to be due to a combination of activation of apoptotic cell-death pathways, release of inflammatory substances such as cytokines, and neuronal excitotoxic effects secondary to excessive glutamate and generation of reactive oxygen and nitrogen species. These secondary mechanisms are the targets of potential therapeutic interventions.

Perinatal hypoxic-ischemic injury is diagnosed clinically by the combination of evidence of fetal distress (heart-rate abnormalities, meconium-stained amniotic fluid), birth depression, and a picture of neonatal encephalopathy. Birth depression is characterized by low Apgar scores at 1 and 5 minutes; in some instances, additional time points are evaluated. The Apgar scores simply reflect the baby's exam findings including: muscle tone and movement in response to stimuli, oxygenation as reflected in the child's skin's color, heart-rate, and respiratory effort. Low Apgar scores and the diagnosis of HIE are usually supported by laboratory studies. Specifically, blood gases may reveal signs of acidosis, and an elevated serum lactate level can be reflective of cellular injury. Upon more detailed examination, neonatal encephalopathy is categorized into three patterns of findings called the Sarnat stages. In some cases, progression can occur from deep stupor or coma in the first 12 hours after injury, to a more hypertonic and jittery presentation at 12–24 hours and again into deeper stages of encephalopathy from 24–72 hours. After approximately 72 hours, the signs of encephalopathy are expected to improve gradually. Many patients with HIE also exhibit seizures shortly after an acute insult. Long or frequent seizures are thought to cause further damage to the brain tissue by creating high metabolic demand on cells that have already endured hypoxic injury. Seizures are most common in the first 48 hours after the injury and they can be either clinical or subclinical.

Since the long-term outcome for asphyxiated infants can be disheartening, prenatal therapeutic interventions have been instituted. Methods used to attempt to lower the risk for HIE include: early and consistent prenatal care, identification and treatment of *in utero* predisposing factors (maternal infection, intrauterine growth retardation, placental abnormalities), and early identification of fetal distress. Once HIE is evident, postnatal interventions are aimed at preventing secondary cellular injury. Currently, the only postnatal intervention with proven benefit for patients who endured HIE is therapeutic hypothermia. Brain cooling is thought to slow cellular metabolism and decrease the inflammation that can cause secondary injury. Cooling protocols have been established at many tertiary care institutions. The protocol should be started within 6 hours of birth. Infants are cooled to a body temperature of 32–33°C, usually for 72 hours. The cooling period is followed by gradual rewarming. The authors of several studies have reported that, as a group, hypothermia-treated patients have decreased rate of death and neurological disability at 18 months of age. Early treatment of HIE is an active area of research, and other therapeutic interventions are forthcoming. Examples of these include intravenous magnesium, erythropoietin, glutamate antagonists, and scavengers of reactive oxygen species.

In patients with HIE, neuroradiological studies help determine the injury's severity. Within the first days, MRI of the brain with diffusion-weighted images (DWI) is the most sensitive test for identifying areas that have endured ischemia and infarction. Two main patterns of injury predominate: cortical (especially parasagittal in the vascular watershed distribution), and deep gray matter (basal ganglia and thalamic) injury. The white matter is often also involved, and less commonly, the brainstem. In addition to abnormalities on the DWI, there may be increased signal on T2-weighted or FLAIR images. As the injury evolves, the test gradually reveals signs of encephalomalacia or loss of brain tissue in the affected areas. The positive diffusion-weighted findings resolve after about one week. Severe basal ganglia involvement or severe diffuse white matter injury are associated with poor clinical outcomes.

EEG findings also help predict the outcome of a child who endures HIE. Aside from specifically helping to identify seizures, the assessment of background electrical activity is helpful. Low amplitude background activity, long intervals between bursts of EEG activity, and absence of sleep-wake cycles by 48 hours are predictive of a poor clinical outcome. A normal and mildly abnormal EEG within 6 hours after birth is usually associated with normal neurodevelopmental outcomes at 24 months of age.

The neurological consequences of HIE can include cerebral palsy, cognitive deficits, and ongoing epilepsy. Recently, there has been recognition of subtle neurodevelopmental abnormalities such as learning disabilities and disorders of behavior, which may not become apparent until preschool or school-age.

Neonatal seizures

A seizure is the manifestation of excessive synchronous electrical neuronal discharges. A clinical seizure is a paroxysmal alteration of neurological function (motor, autonomic, or behavior) as a consequence of the above-mentioned abnormal electrical discharges. An electrographic seizure is considered to have occurred if there are 10 seconds or more of continuous epileptiform discharges on the EEG. Electroclinical dissociation is an uncoupling of the clinical and electrographic expressions of seizures which can lead to an underestimation of true seizure frequency and duration. This last finding is common in premature babies and infants who have been treated with anti-epilepsy medications.

Neonates are particularly vulnerable to seizures on both neuroanatomical and neurophysiological grounds. Ongoing anatomical processes that contribute to seizure susceptibility in the immature brain include: neuronal outgrowth, active synaptogenesis, and deficient myelination. Physiological contributors to seizure vulnerability include the fact that excitatory mechanisms develop prior to inhibitory mechanisms; gamma-amino butyric acid (GABA) being excitatory rather than inhibitory in perinatal neurons; and the absence of a well-developed substantia nigra which would act as part of a seizure inhibitory mechanism. In addition to increased vulnerability, the immature brain is thought to have different mechanisms of seizure generation, propagation, and termination. These factors have contributed to the difficulty in standardizing treatment recommendations.

The seizure types commonly observed in neonates include: clonic (focal or multifocal), tonic (focal), and myoclonic (generalized). Newborns rarely have well-organized, generalized tonic-clonic seizures. A category of seizures unique to the neonatal period is simply referred to as "subtle seizures." These include paroxysmal changes in eye movement, oral-buccal-lingual movements, and apnea. The treatment of seizures in the neonate is based on the etiology of the seizures and the probability of seizure recurrence. In many cases, antiepilepsy medications are prescribed after the first confirmed clinical or electrographic seizure, while the work-up for the etiology of the seizure is in progress. Phenobarbital 20 mg/kg IV is the first line anti-epilepsy medication (AED) for neonatal seizures. Selection of a second and third line AED is inconsistent. As a first step, most clinicians maximize the dose of phenobarbital to 40 mg/kg. If such measure fails to control the events, IV fosphenytoin or levetiracetam are used. Other AEDs used to treat neonates with seizures include benzodiazepines and topiramate. The duration of AED treatment varies from hospital to hospital. As a general rule, AED treatment is continued beyond initial seizure control in patients who have structural brain lesions, infants who required multiple AEDs for seizure control, and patients who have abnormalities in the neurological examination at the time of discharge. A rare form of neonatal onset seizure disorder that is not responsive to AEDs is pyridoxine-dependent seizures. The condition should be suspected in a neonate with medically intractable seizures. In such cases, a therapeutic trial of IV pyridoxine (vitamin B6) should be considered.

With the recognition of electroclinical dissociation, the paradigm has shifted toward considering continuous video-EEG monitoring as the gold standard to aid selecting medications and clinical interventions for patients with neonatal seizures. Use of this technique is recommend for any neonate with documented electrographic seizures, or one who is at high risk for seizures such as those with HIE. Most experts agree that electrographic seizures likely have the same pathophysiology and cause the same sequelae as clinical seizures.

In the neonate, seizures occur in response to acute or sub-acute physiological stress. Examples of such stressors include: HIE, stroke, CNS infection, periventricular and intraventricular hemorrhage, electrolyte abnormalities (hypoglycemia, hypocalcemia, and hypomagnesemia), brain malformations, and inborn errors of metabolism. Laboratory tests that should be considered include quantification of serum glucose, electrolytes, ammonia, lactate, calcium, magnesium, phosphorus, and liver function tests. It is also reasonable to perform a lumbar puncture for the purpose of cerebrospinal fluid analysis. Evaluation of the cerebrospinal fluid should include: cell count, glucose, protein, cerebrospinal fluid bacterial culture, lactate, and amino acids. Finally, a neonate who has seizures needs to undergo neuroradiological evaluation. While MRI of the brain is the preferred modality, obtaining a CT scan or ultrasound of the head, may be more practical.

Twenty-five to thirty-five percent of neonates who endure HIE develop neurological sequelae including mental retardation, motor deficits, and epilepsy. The risk of seizure recurrence in children who are diagnosed with HIE is 10–20%. The odds that a child with HIE will develop epilepsy increase if the child was extremely premature, in the presence of brain malformations, and if the child's EEG background activity has evidence of long interburst intervals and marked voltage suppression.

In utero drug exposure

It goes without saying that exposure to toxins and substances of abuse has a deleterious effect on the fetus. Toxic substance exposure can be evident both in the neonatal period and later in life. The most common substances of abuse that fetuses are exposed to include: alcohol, opiates, cocaine, amphetamines, marijuana, and tobacco.

Alcohol abuse early in gestation can cause abnormalities of the central nervous systems' formation such as microcephaly, neuronal migration defects, and abnormal synapse formation. Poor growth and specific facial features are common in fetal alcohol syndrome. Children exposed to alcohol *in utero* are likely to have long-term problems such as delay in achieving developmental milestones, learning disabilities, attention deficit hyperactivity disorder (ADHD), and other problems of behavior.

Opiate abuse during pregnancy can result in poor growth and low birthweight. Opiate withdrawal (neonatal abstinence syndrome) is probably the most serious complication of maternal opiate abuse. Hyperirritability, tremor, autonomic abnormalities, and seizures can occur in the neonatal period. The authors of several studies have reported that children exposed to opiates *in utero* can later develop ADHD and other behavior problems.

Cocaine exposure *in utero* can cause serious neurological deficits. These include stillbirth, placental abruption, preterm delivery, fetal distress, cerebro-vascular accidents, epilepsy, cerebral palsy, cognitive impairment, and behavior problems.

Methamphetamines exposure *in utero* can increase the risk of premature birth and placental abruption. Long-term consequences are related to hypoxic-ischemic injury.

Marijuana and tobacco exposure *in utero* has been associated with mild neonatal withdrawal syndrome, ADHD, and, later in life, behavior problems.

The hypotonic infant

Hypotonia can be caused by either central (brain, brainstem, and spinal cord) or peripheral (anterior horn cell, peripheral nerves, neuromuscular junction, and muscle) nervous system pathology. Hypotonia may be present at birth or may be identified later in life. Neonatal hypotonia may be a consequence of: hypoxic ischemic injury, especially when the spinal cord is affected; birth trauma; genetic syndromes such as trisomy 21, Prader-Willi syndrome, and leukodystrophies; congenital myotonic dystrophy; spinal muscular atrophy; and transient and congenital forms of myasthenia gravis. Finally, the child may have a disorder referred to as benign congenital hypotonia. This is a diagnosis that can only be made retrospectively, after a child who had unexplained hypotonia spontaneously develops normal muscle tone. The majority of children with benign congenital hypotonia have a central pattern of hypotonia.

Signs and symptoms of hypotonia include: history of decreased fetal movements, breech presentation, arthrogryposis, hip dislocation, respiratory distress, difficulty swallowing (unable to breast feed), excessive drooling, and delay in achieving developmental milestones. At rest, the hypotonic infant does not adopt the expected “fetal posture.” Instead, the child exhibits abduction of the thighs (frog legs). The child’s arms lie at the side of the body with open hands. As would be expected, the hypotonic infant exhibits decreased spontaneous movements. If the infant has had long-standing chest wall weakness, *pectus excavatum* will be observed. Frequently there is flattening of the occiput (plagiocephaly). The hypotonic infant is unable to keep the head upright; when pulled up to a sitting position, the head falls forward. On horizontal suspension, the child’s body drapes over the examiner's hand. And on vertical suspension, the child's head falls forward and the legs dangle.

As is evident, the causes of hypotonia in a neonate are varied. Thus, making diagnostic recommendations is somewhat difficult. The first step in the diagnostic work-up is determining whether the hypotonia is of central or peripheral origin. It is important to recognize that both forms may simultaneously be present. When central origin is suspected, neuroradiological evaluation of the brain and spinal cord is indicated. MRI of the entire neuro-axis is the test of choice. Pathology of peripheral origin can be assessed via: genetic tests, neurophysiological tests (nerve conduction studies, electromyogram), muscle biopsy, nerve biopsy, and tensilon test.

References

Davies JK and Bledsoe JM. Prenatal alcohol and drug exposures in adoption. *Pediatr Clin North Am.* 2005.52:1369–1393.

Edwards AD, Brocklehurst P, Gunn AJ, *et al.* Neurological outcomes at 18 months of age after moderate hypothermia for perinatal hypoxic ischaemic encephalopathy: synthesis and meta-analysis of trial data. *BMJ.* 2010.340:c363.

Fatemi A, Wilson MA, and Johnston M. Hypoxic-ischemic encephalopathy in the term infant. *Clin Perinatol.* 2009.36:835–858.

Fenichel GM. The hypotonic infant. In: Fenichel GM (ed.). *Clinical Pediatric Neurology, A Signs and Symptoms Approach.* 6th ed. Philadelphia: Saunders Elsevier. 2009. pp.153–176.

Glass HC, Wirrell E. Controversies in neonatal seizure management. *J Child Neurol* 2009.24;591–599.

Murray DM, Boylan GB, Ryan CA, *et al.* Early EEG findings in hypoxic-ischemic encephalopathy predict outcomes at 2 years. *Pediatrics.* 2009.124:e459–467.

Perlman JM. Intraventricular hemorrhage and white matter injury in the preterm infant. In: Perlman JM, Polin RA (eds.). *Neurology Neonatology Questions and Controversies.* Philadelphia: Saunders Elsevier. 2008. pp.27–45.

Scher MS. Diagnosis and Treatment of Neonatal Seizures. In: Perlman JM, Polin RA (eds.). *Neurology Neonatology Questions and Controversies.* Philadelphia: Saunders Elsevier. 2008. pp.122–152.

Volpe JJ (ed.). *Neurology of the Newborn*, 5th ed. 2008. Saunders.

21

PALLIATIVE CARE FOR THE PEDIATRIC NEUROLOGIST

Janine Penfield Winters

"You matter because you are you. You matter to the last moment of your life, and we will do all we can, not only to help you die peacefully, but to help you live until you die."

Dame Cicely Saunders

CB was 15 months old when she was diagnosed with infantile onset Batten's disease; her parents were advised that their daughter's life expectancy was 2 to 3 years. Symptoms leading to the diagnosis included seizures, irritability, day–night cycle reversal, blindness, and increasing motor and feeding difficulties. CB's neurologist recommended the surgical insertion of a gastrostomy tube to increase her caloric intake. Her parents were opposed to treatments that would prolong CB's suffering and thus were ambivalent about the feeding tube. At the time CB's diagnosis was confirmed, the family was expecting the birth of a second child. They were informed that each child they bore as a couple had a 25% likelihood of having Batten's disease. In order to help manage these complex discussions, decisions, symptom management and advance care planning, the palliative care service was consulted.

Palliative Care, Nationwide Children's Hospital and The Ohio State University, Columbus, Ohio, USA

Palliative Care Defined

Not all diseases and conditions have a cure. This is particularly true in child neurology, a field in which congenital and degenerative conditions can lead inexorably to a foreshortened life span. Palliative care for the pediatric neurology patient is appropriate for any child whose disease is incurable and will likely lead to death before adulthood. Palliative care is defined as comprehensive, whole person care for both patient and family. Palliative care is not "end of life care." Instead it is a multifaceted approach to prevent and manage suffering for patients for whom a cure is elusive (Figures 1 and 2). Palliative care can be provided concurrently with disease-directed efforts. The child and the family are defined as the unit of care. Palliative care is provided by an interdisciplinary team to expertly address the physical, psychological, social and spiritual aspects of the patients' and families' illness experience, as well as bereavement care. The American Academy of Pediatrics offers the following definition of palliative care:

> *"Palliative care seeks to enhance quality of life and the child's ability to enjoy life in the face of an ultimately terminal condition. The goal is to add life to the child's years, not simply years to the child's life…to optimize the child's experience, rather than hasten death."*

Ideally, the palliative care team is consulted soon after the diagnosis of an incurable condition has been made. The diagnosing physician can introduce the palliative care team as a resource to assist and help guide families when their child is facing a life-limiting or life-threatening condition. Though the disclosure of the diagnosis and prognosis is the responsibility of the child neurologist, members of the palliative care team may be helpful partners during that difficult conversation.

The palliative care team's goals and roles in the care of the patient and family

- Establishing a trusting and longitudinal relationship with the patient/family with special attention to diversity in patient/family needs.
- Caring for the patient and the family throughout the course of an illness with the goal of maximizing comfort for all involved.
- Collaborating with the primary care pediatrician and primary neurologist to assist in decision-making and communication across settings.
- Supporting anticipatory grief (the loss of an expected healthy child).
- Anticipating symptoms that occur near the end-of-life and providing the family with knowledge and tools to address these symptoms.

- Preventing and decreasing suffering by using aggressive measures to control pain and other distressing symptoms.
- Anticipatory guidance and advance care planning in collaboration with the pediatric neurologist.
- Assisting in the establishment of goals of care (as well as specific treatment decisions, as needed) by exploring values, concerns, practical issues and the overall benefits and burdens of proposed treatments with the family.
- Assisting the family and other healthcare providers to re-envision hope.
- Providing supportive care by "sharing the journey."
- Discussing advanced care planning through goal setting and decision making.

The palliative care team established a relationship with CB and her family soon after the diagnosis and provided needed support to CB's family while they awaited genetic testing results for their newborn. The palliative care team worked with CB's parents setting realistic care goals and exploring how treatments, including medically provided nutrition and hydration, fit within these goals. The palliative care team facilitated communication of the family's goals and difficult decisions to the other care providers.

Eliciting concerns

Asking open-ended questions such as "What do you understand about your child's illness?" opens the door for the family to offer their knowledge of the child's condition, their hopes, fears, difficulties, emotional responses, adaptation, or lack thereof. These are often long but necessary conversations. The palliative care team can help elicit this information and partner with the neurologist to facilitate the best care possible for the child and family. Parents' concerns often include fears about symptoms, loss of control, concerns about their family life and financial

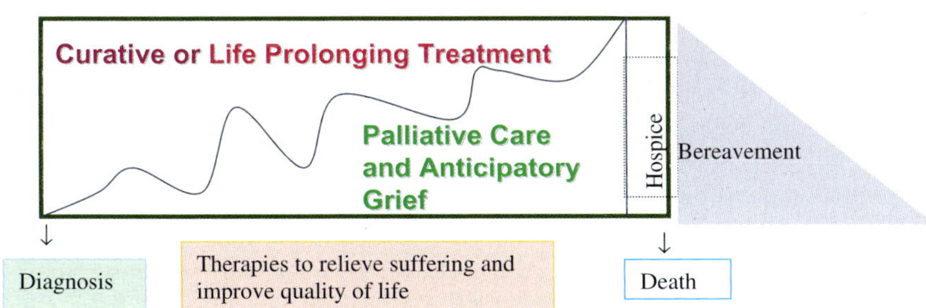

Figure 1. Role of palliative care over the course of an incurable illness.

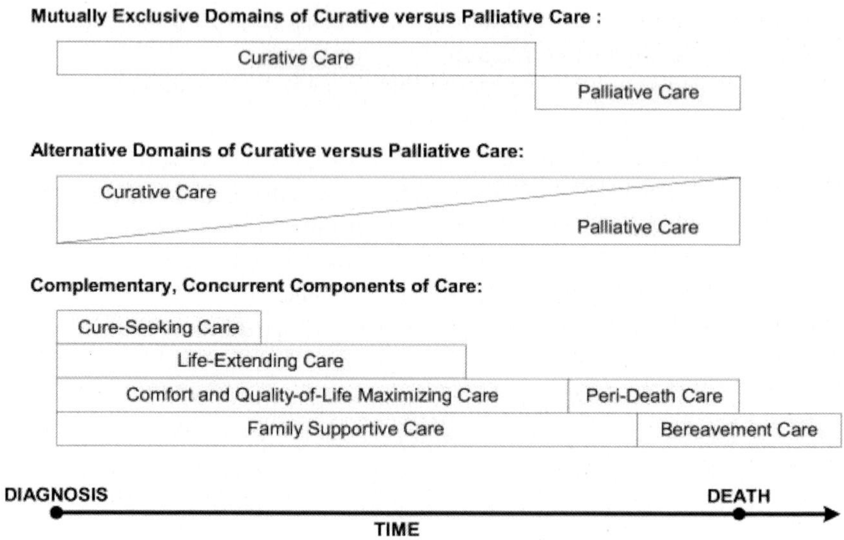

Figure 2. Models for providing pediatric palliative care. Feudtner C *et al. BMC Medicine* 2003;1:3; www.biomedcentral.com.

matters, helping siblings and grandparents cope, fears about the dying process and death itself, spiritual concerns and even doubts. Palliative care teams have the expertise, time and interest to assist families to better understand their situation and to find the means to successfully navigate these difficult waters.

Anticipating Treatment Choices

CB's parents perceived that the child's quality of life was declining, particularly since she had already lost most of her ability to relate to others and experience pleasure. Understanding that her condition was irreversibly worsening, they felt that measures that did not promote CB's comfort were not in her best interest, even if that meant she might survive a shorter time. CB's family was given a multitude of medical intervention choices. After considering the condition from her perspective and as loving parents, they decided that CB would not benefit from the insertion of a feeding tube, but they were interested in pursuing a swallow study to determine if thickening liquids would help prevent aspiration. CB's parents decided to forgo resuscitative attempts and to allow a natural death (AND); formerly DNR (do not resuscitate). Anticipating pulmonary complications, the parents decided to treat CB's infections with oral antibiotics, but would not subject her to the discomfort of

IVs and other invasive procedures. The palliative care team worked with CB's primary and specialty physicians to coordinate communication about treatment decisions.

Anticipating disease progression

Anticipatory guidance about expected symptoms and illness manifestations is particularly important to help parents assess the relative burdens and benefits of treatments prior to critical events. Decision-making in the face of an emergency, when emotions are running high, without advance thought and preparation, is fraught with error and regret. Anticipatory education through the combined efforts and expertise of the neurologist and palliative care team allows families to plan and make informed decisions and to avoid unforseen, and distressing complex bereavement circumstances.

Anticipated complications of degenerative neurological conditions can include: seizures, myoclonus, pain, screaming, loss of milestones, loss of control of oral secretions, swallowing incoordination, aspiration (and resulting recurrent pneumonias), loss of ability to feed orally, weight loss, and loss of normal sleep-wake cycle. Identifying these complications and discussing potential treatment options with parents before they occur, facilitates decision making in alignment with their goals and wishes for the child. Judgment is needed in titrating information flow. These are rarely single conversations. Each individual differs in his or her preference for receiving such information. Sensitivity to personal preferences is important to maintain trust.

While many potential complications of diseases are mentioned above, added attention to respiratory complications is warranted. Respiratory complications are frightening. The parents of children with neurological conditions need to be warned that these complications are virtually inevitable. Parents benefit from counseling that respiratory failure is the usual and expected proximal cause of death for many children with chronic or degenerative neurological conditions. Loss of the ability to manage oral secretions can lead to recurrent pneumonia and irreversible lung damage. Thus, parents need the guidance of the child's neurologist and palliative care team to make decisions about respiratory interventions that best fit their child and family; their choices will change over time with the child's deterioration in health.

The neurologist and the palliative care team can optimally work together to help identify parental wishes related to respiratory complications. Suggested topics for discussion include:

— How to provide pulmonary toilet to prevent pneumonia.
— Whether to allow oral intake for comfort, in the presence of aspiration risk.

— Whether to use oral antibiotics at home for the treatment of pneumonia.
— Using IV antibiotics in the home or hospital for the treatment of pneumonia.
— Non-invasive ventilatory support (CPAP, BiPAP) as a temporary measure.
— Whether to use long-term non-invasive ventilatory support (including risk of facial skin breakdown and of aspiration).
— Whether to use invasive ventilation as a temporary measure (intubation until infections clear, or a time-limited trial of intubation with a plan in case the child cannot be weaned-off mechanical ventilation).
— Whether to consider tracheostomy (balancing recurrent tracheitis, 24-hour tracheostomy care, ongoing risk of mucus plugging and aspiration, inability to hire a babysitter etc.).
— Whether to consider permanent mechanical ventilation for respiratory failure at home or in an institution with the attendant significant consequences for family life and employment).

Managing Symptoms

CB developed several troubling symptoms that her parents identified as uncomfortable. These included: inconsolable crying thought to be due to pain, difficulty swallowing secretions, seizures, day-night cycle reversal, and spasticity. Aggressive management of these distressful symptoms continued over several months to help CB and her family feel more comfortable.

Symptoms: Managing late symptoms in children with incurable neurological disease

While early symptoms of degenerative neurological disorders are often directly related to the brain and neuromuscular systems, late symptoms are often more generalized. Common late symptoms of incurable neurological conditions include: dyspnea, pain, seizures, spasticity, and inability to manage oral secretions. Palliative medicine specialists are trained in aggressive management of symptoms for patients with chronic and serious illnesses as well as those nearing the end of life. Pharmacological interventions often utilized for symptom management can include opioids, NSAIDs, anti-epilepsy medications (for neuropathic pain or seizure control), anti-anxiety medications, antidepressant medications, soporifics, antiemetics, antacids, antipyretics, and occasionally chemotherapy. Complementary therapies that may be of benefit include massage therapy for spasticity, music therapy (especially beneficial for non-verbal children who scream), art therapy and other child-life interventions for the patient and affected siblings. Some parents are interested in complementary/alternative therapies that may have no proven benefit in these conditions, but have little potential for harm. These may include acupuncture/acupressure, hypnosis, biofeedback, energy work (healing touch or Reiki therapy), and prayer. These interventions can help improve the child and the family's quality of life.

Pain and dyspnea are common and distressing symptoms; the treatment of these requires a detailed discussion.

Dyspnea

Adult patients experiencing both dyspnea and pain report that the sensation of air hunger is worse than the pain. In the late phases of many neurological diseases, dyspnea is a common symptom due to recurrent aspiration and pneumonia. Recognition and aggressive treatment of dyspnea or "air hunger" is important in the prevention and relief of suffering. Opioid medications are the most effective treatment for dyspnea. Researchers have shown that opioids, used in correct dosages, do not increase the risk of respiratory depression (Scheme 1).

Pain

This symptom can be divided into nociceptive pain and non-nociceptive pain. Nociceptive pain is caused by stimulation of peripheral nerve fibers that respond to thermal, mechanical and chemical stimulation and is commonly described as aching. Non-nociceptive pain or neuropathic pain is usually described as burning, cold, numbness, "pins and needles", or itching. Neuropathic pain includes dysesthesia and allodynia. Neuropathic pain can be treated with multiple agents including anti-depressants, opioids, anticonvulsants, topicals (lidocaine, capsaicin), NMDA antagonists (ketamine, methadone), cannabinoids, corticosteroids, baclofen, TENS units, acupuncture and other modalities. As a general rule, opioids and non-opioid treatments work better together than either one alone. Nociceptive pain includes visceral, deep somatic and superficial somatic pain. In the presence of nociceptive pain, there should be prompt oral administration of medications in the following order: non-opioids (e.g. acetaminophen); then, as necessary, mild opioids, then strong opioids such as morphine until the patient is free of pain. The World Health Organization's (WHO) "pain ladder" is a worldwide accepted standard which guides medical providers on how to manage nociceptive pain (Figure 3).

WHO's pain treatment guidelines recommend a round-the-clock treatment for chronic pain. To maintain freedom from pain, long-acting medications should

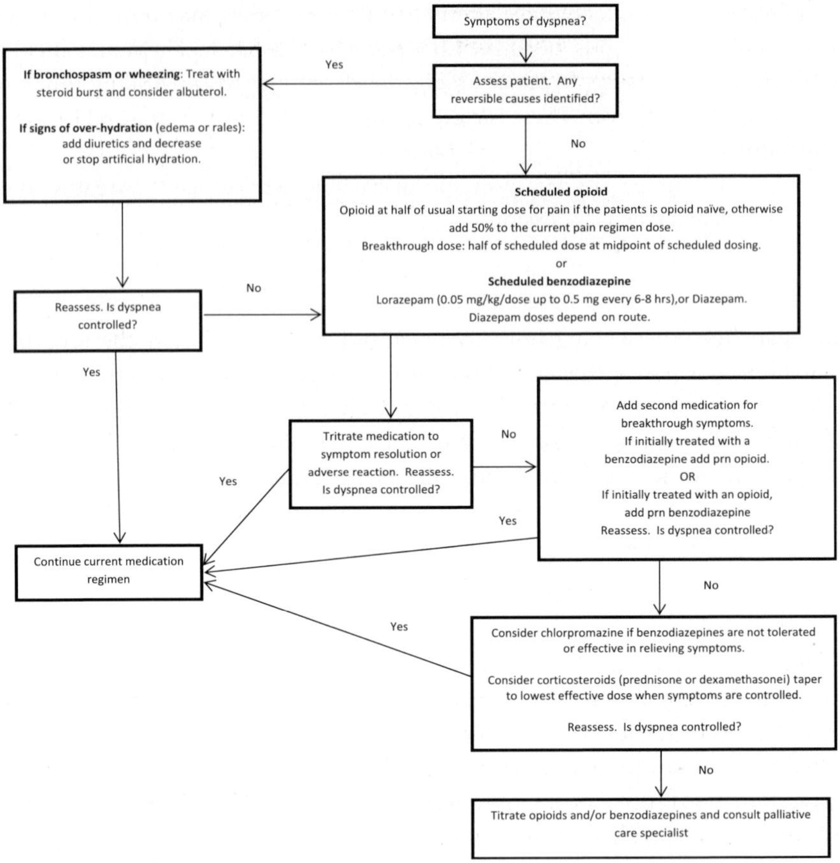

Scheme 1. Medication management of acute dyspnea.

Notes:

1. Burst steroid dosing: Prednisone 1–2 mg/kg/day in two divided doses; max 60 mg/day for 3–10 days; Prednisolone and Methylprednisolone dosing is the same as Prednisone.
2. Dexamethasone 0.6 mg/kg × 1 dose (max 16 mg).
3. Do not use Methadone for dyspnea.
4. In opioid-naïve children (>6 months of age), start with oral morphine equivalent of 0.2–0.3 mg/kg/dose up to 2.5 mg q 4h. If already on opioids, add half the scheduled 4-hr dose for breakthrough q 1 hr PRN.
5. If renal insufficiency, substitute oxycodone for morphine due to lower risk of accumulation of toxic metabolites.

be prescribed "by the clock," rather than "on demand." Additionally, immediate release medications should be prescribed for "breakthrough" pain. In general, immediate release medications should be 5–15% of the total daily baseline dose of long-acting medication (Scheme 2). WHO's pain relief ladder is designed to

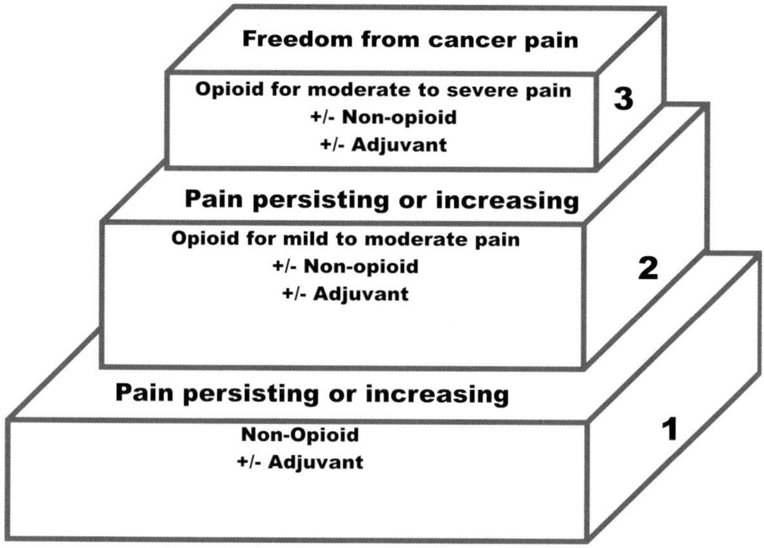

Figure 3. WHO pain relief ladder.

provide the "right drug in the right dose at the right time" in a cost-effective manner, providing 80–90% efficacy of achieving pain control. In children with severe neurological disability, medications may need to be available in concentrates for oral administration, preparations that can be administered via gastrostomy tubes, or occasionally IV or subcutaneous preparations. Studies have been performed with long-acting opioid preparations in sprinkle form, and these can be administered successfully via gastrostomy tubes.

All medications, including opioids, have anticipatable side effects or adverse drug reactions (ADRs). Allergies to opioids are rare and consist of hives, wheezing or cardiovascular collapse; itching alone does not constitute an allergy. Children and their parents tolerate opioids ADRs poorly if not forewarned and if there is no plan in place. The six common ADRs for opioids and their solutions are:

1. Itching. Solution: Have antihistamines available as initial itching usually is due to opioid-induced histamine release.
2. Nausea. Solution: Usually resolves in 2–3 days on the same dose, consider dopamine receptor blocker.
3. Sedation. Solution: Usually resolves in 2–3 days on the same dose, counseling that catch-up sleep is expected for patients who have not slept well recently.
4. Urinary retention. Solution: Consider temporary urinary catheter, also may resolve spontaneously.

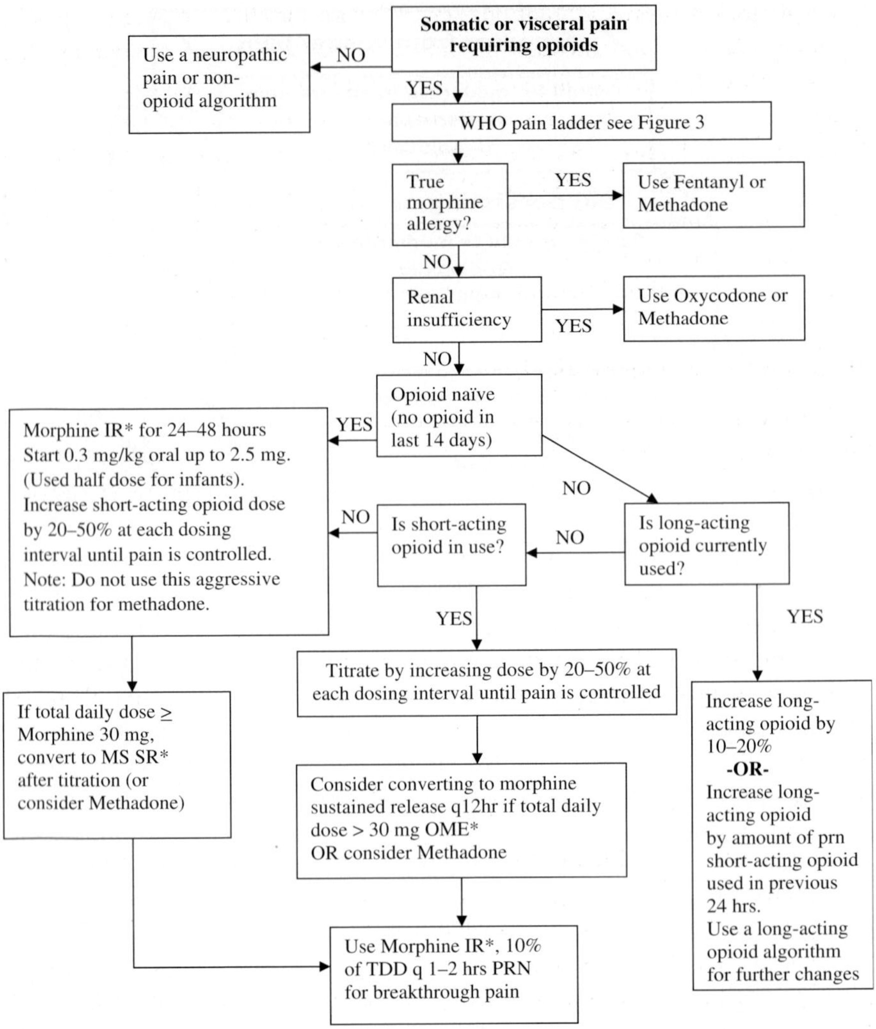

* OME – Oral morphine equivalent
* IR – Immediate release
* SR – Sustained release

Scheme 2. Pediatric somatic/visceral pain management algorithm for opioids. *Notes*: Morphine liquid (20 mg/ml) or tablets are cost-effective and standard first choice for breakthrough pain. Other opioids can be substituted (check conversion tables).

5. Respiratory depression. Solution: Start with lowest effective dose of opioids. Often resolves spontaneously in hours to days. Counsel the family that respiratory depression happens gradually and that respiratory depression is always accompanied by depressed mentation and poor arousability.
6. Constipation. Solution: All patients on opioids should receive laxatives and stool softeners with adjustments based on bowel movement volume, consistency and frequency. This side effect does not resolve with time. This side effect is of particular concern in neurologically impaired individuals due to underlying condition, poor fluid intake and decreased activity level.

Titrating opioid pain medications

Table 1 provides starting doses for pain control in opioid-naïve patients. The table lists methods for titrating daily opioid doses and breakthrough doses for the patient with continuing pain. Additionally, the medical provider must consider if the patient is having incident pain (pain that is situation-specific or time-limited). If the patient is experiencing incident pain, there should not be an escalation of titration of routine daily doses of long-acting pain medications, but immediate release breakthrough medications should be provided in anticipation of the activity (e.g. before physical therapy sessions). Table 2 provides equi-analgesic doses when changing from one opioid to another or changing route of administration.

End-of-life care planning: Decisions about resuscitation effects

Planning for the end of life is not a one-time "get the code status" conversation. A provider who has an ongoing relationship with the family can help them determine the best choices for the child. Often, parents will state their wish for a cure or miracle. This should not be taken as a conversation stopper — it is truly what parents wish, hope, or pray for. That does not mean they do not have a very realistic idea of their child's prognosis and impending death. It is a sign of empathy to affirm the parents' hopes, while at the same time discussing realistic goals and options based on what the medical team and family can control. Conversations with the family about options are more likely to be perceived as helpful if the medical team has learned about the family's unique values and the cultural and religious contexts in which they make decisions (Figure 4). Important items to address when the child is nearing the end-of-life include:

— What are the goals, the benefits and the burdens of intubation, CPR, or cardiac defibrillation?

Table 1. Starting dose of medications for pain control in opioid-naïve patients.

Medication	Starting dose for opioid naïve patient in pain	Criteria for dose increase	Size of titration increase, all titrations at next scheduled dose	Breakthrough (BT) dose titration
Morphine immediate release (Avoid/reduce for renal failure)	PO/SL/PR: 0.15–0.3 mg/kg every 4 hrs (up to adult dose) and prn dose 0.1–0.15 mg/kg q1h prn Subc/IV: 0.05–0.1 mg/kg every 4 hrs + 0.05 mg/kg q1h prn	Increase if current dose ineffective as demonstrated by three or more BT doses in 24 hrs for breakthrough pain	PO/SL/PR: Increase by 0.15 mg/kg mg per dose up to 10 mg; > than 10 mg/dose, increase by 50%. Subc/IV: double dose up to 1 mg; > than 1 mg/dose, increase by 50%.	Increase breakthrough doses proportionally with dose, BT dose can be ½ of scheduled dose OR 10% of total daily dose
Morphine sustained release (Not appropriate in patients with renal failure)	Not recommended in opioid naïve patients: lowest dose = 15 mg every 12 hrs	Increase if current dose ineffective as demonstrated by three or more BT doses in 24 hrs for breakthrough pain	Increase by 50% of previous dose (increase 15 mg or other doses from q 12 hrs to q 8 hrs or in doses higher than 15 mg/dose, increase dose by 50% at same interval)	Increase breakthrough doses proportionally with dose, BT dose can be ½ of scheduled dose OR 10% of total daily dose
Oxycodone immediate release	0.1–0.2 mg/kg every 4 hrs 0.05–0.1 mg/kg q1h prn	Increase if current dose ineffective as demonstrated by three or more BT doses in 24 hrs for breakthrough pain	Increase by 0.1 mg/kg for dose up to 10 mg; > than 10 mg/dose, increase by 50%	Increase breakthrough doses proportionally with dose, BT dose can be ½ of scheduled dose OR 10% of total daily dose

(*Continued*)

Table 1. *(Continued)*

Medication	Starting dose for opioid naïve patient in pain	Criteria for dose increase	Size of titration increase, all titrations at next scheduled dose	Breakthrough (BT) dose titration
Oxycodone sustained release	Not recommended in opioid naïve patients: Lowest dose = 10 mg every 12 hrs	Increase if current dose ineffective as demonstrated by three or more BT doses in 24 hrs for breakthrough pain	Increase by 50% of previous doses (increase 10 mg or other doses from q 12 hrs to q 8 hrs or in doses higher than 10 mg/dose, increase dose by 50% at same interval)	Increase breakthrough doses proportionally with dose, BT dose can be ½ of scheduled dose OR 10% of total daily dose
Combination product: Oxycodone + acetaminophen	0.1–0.2 mg/kg q 4 hrs APAP dose 10–15 mg/kg/dose. Adult starting doses: ½ of 5/325 (for patients > 25 kg) Liquid: O/APAP 5/325 per 5ml (Roxicet)-contains 0.5% ethanol	Increase if current dose ineffective	Titrate as acetaminophen content allows (3) APAP Max: < 2 yrs: 60 mg/kg/day 2–12 yrs: 75 mg/kg/day, not to exceed 3750 mg/day	Used often as BT dose with close tracking of total daily acetaminophen dose
Hydromorphone	PO/SL/PR: 0.05 mg/kg every 4 hrs + 0.025 mg/kg q1h prn Subc/IV: 0.025-0.075 mg/kg every 3–4 hrs + 0.025 mg q1h	Increase if current dose ineffective as demonstrated by three or more BT doses in 24 hrs for breakthrough pain	PO/SL/PR: Increase the dose by 0.025 mg up to 4 mg; > than 4 mg/dose, increase by 50%. Subc/IV: Increase by 0.025 mg/kg for dose up to 1 mg; > than 1 mg/dose, increase by 50%	Increase breakthrough doses proportionally with dose, BT dose can be ½ of scheduled dose OR 10% of total daily dose

(Continued)

Table 1. (*Continued*)

Medication	Starting dose for opioid naïve patient in pain	Criteria for dose increase	Size of titration increase, all titrations at next scheduled dose	Breakthrough (BT) dose titration
Combination Product: Hydrocodone + Acetaminophen (H/APAP)	0.1–0.2 mg/kg q 4 hrs APAP dose 10–15 mg/kg/dose. Adult starting doses: half 5/325 tab (for patients > 25 kg). Don't start with 7.5 mg tab. Liquid: H/APAP 7.5 mg/325 mg per 15 ml and 10 mg/325 mg per 15 ml solutions, contain about 7% ethanol	Increase if current dose ineffective	Titrate as acetaminophen content allows (3). APAP max: < 2 yrs: 60 mg/kg/day 2–12 yrs: 75 mg/kg/day, not to exceed 3750 mg/day	Used often as BT dose with close tracking of total daily acetaminophen dose
Methadone	Extreme caution in opioid naïve. Request expert advice. Adult starting dose 2.5 mg/dose BID.	If breakthrough doses are needed more than two times per day to treat baseline pain, consider methadone dose increase by 10–25%	Titration frequency no more than every 3–4 days. Methadone dose increase by 10–30%[4]	Do not use methadone for breakthrough pain.

(*Continued*)

Table 1. (*Continued*)

Medication	Starting dose for opioid naïve patient in pain	Criteria for dose increases	Size of titration increase, all titrations at next scheduled dose	Breakthrough (BT) dose titration
Codeine & codeine combination products	Not recommended due to genetic variability in metabolism to active metabolite morphine (4)			

Citation/Notes:

(1) PO: oral; SL: sublingual; PR: rectal; AAP: acetaminophen; PRN: on demand; SUBC: subscutaneous; BT: breakthrough; BID: twice a day.

(2) Pediatric and Neonatal Lexi-Drugs Online. Hudson (OH): Lexi-Comp, Inc. 2010. http://www.crlonline.com.

(3) Changes in dosage forms available for APAP based on FDA action will be in effect January 2014 — no more than 325 mg of APAP in any prescription combination product per dose. Manufacturers are starting to change formulations now so availability in the coming months of the 500 mg, 650 mg, and 750 mg combo products will become scarce/unavailable in anticipation of the 2014 deadline. http://www.fda.gov/Drugs/DrugSafety/ucm239821.htm.

(4) Williams DG, Patel A, Howard RF. Pharmacogenetics of codeine metabolism in an urban population of children and its implications for analgesic reliability. *Br J Anaesth* 2002;89:839–845.

Table 2. Opioids: Equianalgesic doses, duration of action[1].

Generic name	Examples of trade names	SC, IV	Oral	Rectal	Duration of action (hrs)
	Recommended for chronic pain management				
Morphine sulfate	Roxanol	10 mg	30 mg	30 mg	4[3,5]
Hydromorphone	Dilaudid	1.5 mg	4.5 mg[2]	4.5 mg [2]	3–4[3,6]
Oxycodone	Roxicodone; in combination with ASA or Acetaminophen[4,5]: Percocet, Percodan, Roxicet, Tylox	–	20 mg	20 mg	4
Hydrocodone	In combination with ASA or Acetaminophen[4]: Vicodin, Lortab, Lorcet	–	30 mg	30 mg	4
Methadone[7]		Use a Methadone dosing protocol			
Transdermal fentanyl	Duragesic transdermal patch	180–200 mg oral morphine per 24 hrs = 100 mcg/hour transdermal fentanyl applied every 72 hrs. Onset of action 12–24 hrs, ensure adequate analgesia during this time by providing additional short-acting opioid for PRN use. Fentanyl absorption varies with weight loss (decreased absorption) and fever (increased absorption)			

(*Continued*)

Table 2. (*Continued*)

NOT RECOMMENDED for chronic pain management: codeine, butarphanol, levorphanol, meperidine, nalbuphine, and penfazocin

Citation/Notes:
1. Consider reducing calculated dose by 1/3–1/2 when changing from oral to parenteral, transdermal to any other route, or from one opioid to another to accommodate for incomplete cross sensitivity, absorption variability, and patient variability.
2. Expert sources disagree about hydromorphone conversion, 4.5 mg = 30 Oral Morphine Equivalents (OME) and 7.5 mg = 30 mg OME are both used.
3. Oral route provides the longest duration of action.
4. Use current recommendations for maximum dose of acetaminophen per 24 hrs.
5. Sustained release morphine and oxycodone should not be given any more frequently than every 8–12 hrs.
6. Suggested initial dosage intervals for oral/SQ = q 4hrs IV = q 3hrs.
7. Recommended methadone dosing should be reviewed with clinical pharmacist and dosed by a protocol.
8. Codeine is not recommended due to genetic variability of metabolism to the active metabolite, i.e. Morphine. Slow metabolizers do not achieve pain relief and rapid metabolizers are prone to overdose complications.

American Pain Society "Principles of Analgesic Use in the Treatment of Acute Pain and Cancer Pain." 5th Ed. 2003.
Primer of Palliative Care, 4th Edition, Ohio Pain Initiative, Analgesic table, 2007. www.ohiopaininitiative.org

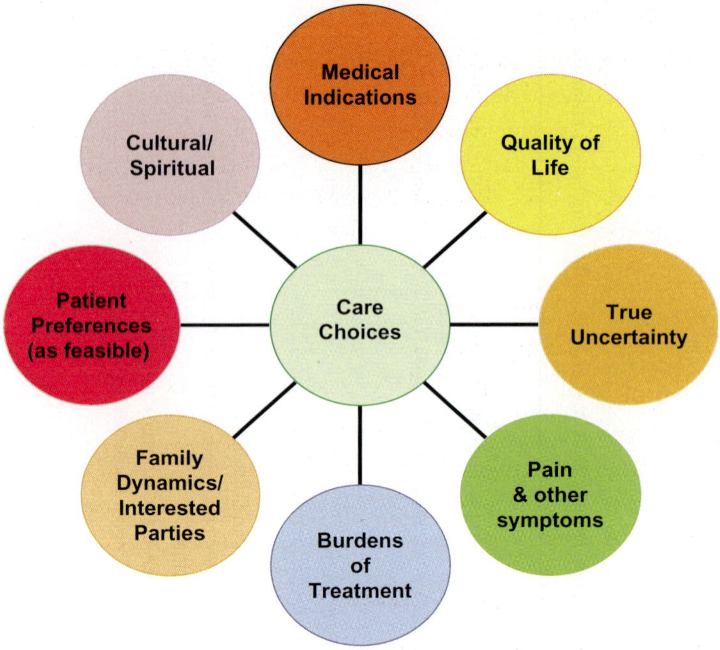

Figure 4. Key elements for decision-making about resuscitation measures.

— How would intubation, CPR, cardiac defibrillation and ICU admission benefit or harm the patient and family, both in the short and longer term? What is the likely outcome?
— How would intubation, CPR, cardiac defibrillation and ICU admission affect the patient's duration and quality of life?
— If survival is possible, what does that look like for the patient and the family?
— If they choose not to pursue attempts at resuscitation, what plans will be made to ensure a peaceful death (e.g. out-of-hospital DNR orders, coordination with hospice, school, EMS, extended family and neighbors, counseling of siblings and symptom control measures).

Focus on ethics

Will interventions such as intubation, CPR, or cardiac defibrillation help the patient, or cause undue suffering or harm? Will resuscitation comply with the ethical principles of beneficence, non-maleficence, autonomy, and justice?

Focus on a natural process

Use neutral language such as "Allow Natural Death" to express the idea that death is a normal part of the lifecycle and that prolonging the dying process using medical technology may not provide benefit. Using the terms "heroic" or "life-sustaining" to describe invasive and non-beneficial interventions unfairly biases the parents towards accepting ICU care that they may otherwise reject when considering their child's best interests.

Focus on continuing to work together

Avoid language that implies abandonment such as "we cannot do anything else" or "withdrawing care." Focus on what the team can do to alleviate suffering such as supporting the family through their crisis or promoting meaningful memories. Help families know they will receive personalized care and treatments to ensure the best outcome for the child and family even as the end of life approaches.

Focus on identifying what the family can control

The care team can help the family control the place of death (home, ICU, hospice room), who is present, level of comfort, memory-making (handprints, pictures), and sometimes fulfilling a last wish.

Focus on sharing the moral burden

The physician's essential role is to make recommendations based on his or her medical knowledge and clinical experience. Most laymen have minimal knowledge on which to base medical decisions. Most families have limited experience with complex illness and death — especially when the patient is a child. When a child is dying, it is important not to imply that there is a choice to be made about whether or not he dies. This is unfair to parents who may then live with the perception and associated guilt that they have played a role in the child's death. This often leads to complicated bereavement. For example, signing a "Do Not Resuscitate (DNR) form" can in time feel like having "signed the child's death warrant." In many American states, parents do not have to sign a "DNR form." Instead, a physician signs the document after a family meeting in which decisions are made together; record of that conversation is entered into the medical chart.

CB's parents worked with the palliative care team to find new hope — they identified aspects of CB's experiences of life and dying that they could make better. CB's parents received guidance and chose how they wanted the child cared for at the end of life, and where they preferred for her to die. After 20 months of slow but noticeable clinical decline, CB began a phase of rapid deterioration, becoming less responsive and unable to eat from a spoon or suck on her bottle. This culminated in the inability to swallow. CB's parents called their Home Hospice team — the nurse, chaplain and social worker each responded to their needs and questions, making daily visits to their home. Several days later, CB died peacefully in her sleep, at home, and in her own bed.

Death is one moment in time. The rest is living.

Physical Changes in the Final Hours of Life

Thus far, we have focused on improving the quality of life of patients and families affected by serious neurological conditions. Palliative care teams are most effective in the weeks, months or even years before death. That said, nurses and physicians experienced in palliative care have particular expertise in anticipating and recognizing the expected physical changes close to the end of life, which will be the focus of the remainder of this chapter.

The medical team should provide the family anticipatory guidance on the physical changes expected at the end of life. Understanding those changes can prevent emotional distress and family crises. Many physical changes at the end of life do not need to be treated, unless the patient appears to be uncomfortable. Not all of the following will occur in any one patient, but these symptoms are all common in the final hours of life.

Neurological changes

Decreased level of consciousness, somnolence, agitation/terminal delirium, difficulty swallowing, loss of sphincter control, changes in respiration, and difficulty controlling body temperature.

Gastrointestinal changes

Decreased appetite, difficulty swallowing, difficulty managing secretions, loss of gag reflex, decreased gastrointestinal motility. Nausea and emesis are likely to occur if the patient is fed artificially as the gastrointestinal tract begins to fail. Hunger cannot be experienced by unconscious individuals.

Pulmonary changes

Decreased tidal volume, episodes of apnea, increased work of breathing, Cheyne-Stokes breathing, and "death rattle."

Integumentary changes

Mottling or cyanosis. Skin breakdown may occur due to either fragility of the skin or poor healing as nutritional status deteriorates.

Cardiovascular changes

Rhythm changes, hypotension, peripheral cooling, cyanosis and mottling. Distal extremity edema is a common sign in the young child who is close to death.

It is important for both the family and providers to understand the differences between normal changes of the body (as it nears death), "symptoms" and "suffering." The normal changes of the body are described above. If these changes are noticed as uncomfortable by the patient (and to some extent, the family), they qualify as symptoms and the patient or family should be offered treatments. Suffering is experienced by conscious beings, not their bodies. By definition, therefore, unconscious individuals cannot experience suffering, though their families can. The construct of suffering is much broader than physical, and encompasses existential, spiritual, social, practical (including financial), and emotional concerns for patients and their loved ones. Prevention and treatment of suffering is the defining feature of palliative care.

Recognition and Treatment of Suffering by the Interdisciplinary Team

Team members such as social workers, chaplains, child life specialists, nurses and others working together can best recognize the roles of the following types of pain contributing to the patient's suffering:

- Physical pain: pain due to disease or its treatment and residual effects.
- Social pain: isolation from loved ones and familiar environs, estrangement.
- Spiritual/existential pain: "why me?"; protective silence (protecting parents); moral burden "have I left a mark on the world, will I be forgotten?"
- Psychological pain: fear, anxiety, guilt, anger.
- Need to leave a legacy — for instance — physical legacy: such as pictures, handprints, footprints or lock of hair.

While not all suffering is physical, medication management may be beneficial for many common symptoms including dyspnea, pain, anxiety/agitation, nausea, emesis, constipation, and excessive secretions. If a conscious patient does not achieve relief as expected from pain medications, other forms of suffering may be contributing to the perception of pain. For an excellent discussion of suffering and the Hospice and Palliative Care philosophy, please read "UNIPAC One: The Hospice/Palliative Approach to End-of-Life Care" (available at www.aahpm.org).

Preventing Distressing Symptoms at the End of Life

Medical providers sometimes fail to recognize the terminal phase of illness and may provide interventions at the end of life that, though well-intended, increase patients' suffering. The following is a discussion of clinical pearls to recognize to avoid suffering at the end of life.

Avoid medically provided nutrition/hydration near the end of life. The gastrointestinal tract is beginning to fail and patients rarely feel hunger or thirst. Artificial feeding in the final hours and days of life frequently causes GI discomfort, distention, nausea, and emesis. The natural process just before death is that dehydration is common. Dehydration is well tolerated and is observed to be more comfortable than complications of artificial hydration (increased oral-nasal secretions, pulmonary and integumentary edema leading to dyspnea and skin breakdown).

Avoid overhydration near the end of life. Medical hydration near the end of life increases secretions that a patient cannot manage (increases "death rattle"). Medical hydration is difficult to titrate near the end of life as the renal and cardiovascular systems begin to fail. Excess fluid accumulates in the lungs and under the skin. Furosemide will no longer reverse overhydration in the context of renal shut-down just before death. Thus, hydration near the end of life often causes difficult-to-manage pulmonary edema and dyspnea. A long-standing medical pearl dictates "It is better to die dry than to die wet."

When adequate education is provided, families understand and usually accept limiting the risk of harm from medical nutrition and hydration at the end of life. One suggestion is to counsel families "IV fluids do not go where they will help the patient, the fluid collects in the lungs and skin of a patient whose body is shutting down." Helping families to understand their child is not experiencing hunger or thirst if unconscious and thus they are not "starving" or abandoning their child in any way can be helpful to them as they (and many healthcare providers) struggle with the concept. Mouth care is essential in this phase of the dying process as well.

Grief and bereavement

After a child under the neurologist's care dies, the minimum role for the primary neurologist is to refer the family to a bereavement program, to send condolence cards and to call the family at least once. Access to a quality bereavement program is an important reason for every child with a terminal illness to be involved with a palliative care program. Palliative care programs often receive feedback from families that continuous support through the entire 25-month bereavement period has provided the most memorable positive impact on the family. For a childhood death, an extended bereavement program (25 months) is ideal. This period is 1 year longer than the typical adult bereavement program because of the nature of childhood loss. The second year after death of a child can be more difficult for parents than the first year. A bereavement program ideally addresses the needs of parents, siblings, grandparents, community and healthcare providers.

Conclusion

Perhaps someday neurological diseases that are currently irreversible and terminal will have a cure. In the meantime, palliative care can provide longitudinal assistance to neurologists who are trying to meet patients' and families' needs. Services provided by a palliative care team can include intensive symptom management, support for the patient and family during their illness experience, coordinated communication, and goal-setting. The longitudinal relationship with the patient and family is critical. Said relationship helps maximize the effectiveness of palliative care, by assisting families to develop individualized coping strategies, find meaning, maintain hope and make decisions contextualized to their unique situation, cultural and religious preferences.

Recommended Resources

American Academy of Hospice and Palliative Medicine (www.aahpm.org)
World Health Organization Pain Relief Ladder
AAHPM UNIPAC One: The Hospice Palliative Medicine Approach to End-of-Life Care. Third Edition.

AAHPM UNIPAC Eight: The Hospice and Palliative Medicine Approach to Caring for Pediatric Patients. 3rd ed.

"My Wishes" a booklet from www.agingwithdignity.org for thought provoking questions that allow effective advance care planning

References

Anesthesia Online: http://priory.com/anaes/neuropathic.htm

Clemens KE, Klaschik E. Symptomatic therapy of dyspnea with strong opioids and its effect on ventilation in palliative care patients. *J Pain Symptom Manage.* 2007.33:473–481.

Clemens KE, Quednau I, Klaschik E. Is there a higher risk of respiratory depression in opioid-naïve palliative care patients during symptomatic therapy of dyspnea with strong opioids? *J Palliat Med.* 2008.11:204–216.

Eisenberg E, McNicol ED, Carr DB. Opioids for neuropathic pain. Cochrane Database of Systematic Reviews 2006, Issue 3. Art. No.: CD006146. DOI: 10.1002/14651858.CD006146 http://www2.cochrane.org/reviews/en/ab006146.html

Harlos, M. Symptom Management In Comfort End-of-Life Care of Pneumonia. http://palliative.info/resource_material/Pneumonia_EOL.pdf

Keskinbora K, Pekel AF, Aydinli I. Gabapentin and an opioid combination versus opioid alone for the management of neuropathic cancer pain: a randomized open trial. *J Pain Symptom Manage.* 2007.34:183–189.

Raja SN, Haythornthwaite JA. Combination therapy for neuropathic pain — which drugs, which combination, which patients? *N Engl J Med.* 2005.352:1373–1375.

22

TIC DISORDER AND TOURETTE SYNDROME

Pedro Weisleder and Latif Khuhro

The neurology consultant evaluates an 8-year-old boy for the chief complaint of frequent eye blinking and throat clearing. The child's mother indicates the boy's frequent eye blinking began 8 months prior to the visit. During the school week, the child's frequent eye blinking is incessant; the symptom improves on weekends. In addition, 3 months before the visit, the child began clearing his throat — even when he was not experiencing an upper respiratory tract infection. On further questioning, the child's mother describes the boy as "fidgety, unable to sit still." Evaluation by an ophthalmologist and an otolaryngologist were not fruitful. The child's pediatrician indicated the boy's symptoms are most likely tics. The mother wants to know what tics are and how they relate to Tourette syndrome.

Tic Disorder

Tics are sudden, brief, purposeless, nonrhythmic, stereotyped, repetitive, involuntary movements (motor tics) or vocalizations (vocal tics). Eighty percent of the tics involve the face; 69% the neck; 55% the upper extremities; and 26% the lower

Division of Child Neurology, Nationwide Children's Hospital and The Ohio State University, Columbus, Ohio, USA

extremities. The movements and vocalizations can be classified as either simple or complex. Examples of simple motor tics are frequent eye blinking, facial grimacing, nose twitching, shoulder shrugging, and head shaking. Common vocal tics include humming, throat clearing, and grunting. Complex motor tics are distinct and coordinated patterns of movements involving several muscle groups. These include jumping, kicking, stamping, or ritualistically performing a series of movements. Some tics are so severe they lead to self injury such as: head banging, orifice digging, and self-biting. Finally, the following are examples of complex vocal tics: singing, whistling, echolalia (repeating other people's utterances), and palilalia (repeating one's utterances).

Tics are more common in children, where one in four have a tic during the school years. Tic disorders tend to occur in families, and are five times more common in boys than girls. Tic onset is usually between the ages of 3 and 8 years. Nine out of ten children who have tics will experience significant symptom improvement by the time they reach adulthood. People who exhibit tics report what are described as premonitory urges — the need to perform a tic in order to relieve the urge or decrease the sensation. Although tics are involuntary, some people can occasionally suppress, camouflage, or otherwise manage their tics in an effort to minimize their impact on functioning. It is well known that tic frequency and severity fluctuate with time. In addition, the severity of tics increases during periods of anxiety, stress, and fatigue. Conversely, it is generally accepted that sleep, rest, and being focused on an activity lessen tic severity. Some medications such as psychoactive drugs may increase tic severity. A patient who exhibits tics, where the symptoms last less than one year, is said to have a transient tic disorder. Tics are the most frequent, although not the only, symptom of Tourette syndrome.

Tourette Syndrome

Tourette syndrome (TS) is a disorder characterized by the presence of tics and other neuropsychological symptoms. The disorder is named after Dr. Georges Gilles de la Tourette, a French neurologist, who described the condition in 1885. For a patient to be diagnosed as having TS, they have to exhibit one or more motor and vocal tic for at least one year. During this period there is no tic-free period of more than 3 consecutive months. Symptom onset is prior to age 18 years. And the symptoms are not caused by a substance or medication, or by another medical condition. Neuropsychological conditions that are often associated to TS include: impulsivity, explosive behavior, attention deficit and attention deficit-hyperactivity disorder (ADD or ADHD), obsessive-compulsive behaviors, and learning difficulties. As would be expected given the natural history of tics, the early symptoms of TS are first noticed in childhood. TS occurs in people from all ethnic backgrounds.

As previously mentioned, tics come and go over time, varying in type, frequency, location, and severity. The first symptoms usually occur in the head and neck area and may progress to include muscles of the trunk and extremities. Motor tics generally precede the development of vocal tics, and simple tics often precede complex tics. Most patients experience peak tic severity before the end of puberty. Symptom improvement for the majority of patients occurs during the late teen years and early adulthood. Approximately 10% of those with TS have a progressive or disabling course that lasts into adulthood. Although the disorder is genereally lifelong and chronic, it is not a degenerative condition. Individuals with TS have a normal life expectancy. TS does not impair intelligence. The precise cause and anatomical substrate of tic disorder and TS is unknown. Researchers, however, point at abnormalities in brain regions where dopaminergic and serotoninergic neurons interact. These include the striatum, substantial nigra, thalamus, and prefrontal cortex. But given the complex presentation of TS, the cause of the disorder is likely to be equally complex.

Conditions related to TS

As indicated above, tics are but one symptom of TS. Patients with TS also experience neuropsychological problems including inattention, hyperactivity, impulsivity, learning problems, and obsessive-compulsive symptoms. The latter are exemplified by worries about dirt and germs which are associated with repetitive hand-washing. Similarly, patients with obsessive-compulsive thoughts may exhibit ritualistic behaviors such as counting, repeating, or ordering and arranging. People with TS have also reported problems with depression and anxiety that may or may not be directly related to TS.

Diagnosis of TS

The diagnosis of TS is made on clinical grounds. That is, the patient needs to meet the clinical criteria described above. There are no blood or laboratory tests needed for the diagnosis of TS. That said, neuroimaging studies (MRI of brain, CT scan of the head), electroencephalogram (EEG), and certain blood tests may be used to rule out other conditions that might be confused with TS. It is not uncommon for patients to be formally diagnosis as having TS only after symptoms have been present for some time. The reasons for this are many. For families and physicians unfamiliar with TS, mild and even moderate tic symptoms may be considered inconsequential, part of a developmental phase, or the result of another condition.

For example, parents may think that eye blinking is related to vision problems or that sniffling is related to seasonal allergies. Many patients are self-diagnosed after they, their parents, other relatives, or friends read or hear about TS.

Treatment of TS

In the majority of patients, the symptoms of TS are mild. For that reason, most physicians tend not to prescribe medications for the condition. That said, and given the range of potential complications, people with TS are best served by receiving medical care from a multidisciplinnary team who can offer a comprehensive treatment plan.

Medications

Effective medications are available for those with TS whose symptoms interfere with functioning. Neuroleptics are the class of medications most commonly used for tic suppression; a number are available but some are more effective than others. Unfortunately, there is no one medication that is helpful to all people with TS, nor does any medication completely eliminate symptoms. In addition, all medications have side effects. Treatment decisions must include a risk/benefit analysis balancing the potential for side effects against the benefit to the patient. The side effects of most neuroleptic medications can be managed by initiating treatment slowly and reducing the dose as soon as side effects occur. The most common side effects of neuroleptics include sedation, weight gain, and cognitive dulling. Neurological side effects such as tremor, dystonic reactions (twisting movements or postures), parkinsonian-like symptoms, and other dyskinetic (involuntary) movements are less common and are readily managed with dose reduction. Discontinuing neuroleptics after long-term use must be done slowly to avoid rebound increases in tics and withdrawal dyskinesias. One form of withdrawal dyskinesia called tardive dykinesia is a movement disorder distinct from TS that may result from the chronic use of neuroleptics. The risk of this side effect can be reduced by using lower doses of neuroleptics for shorter periods of time. A list of neuroleptic medications commonly used for the treatment of tics is presented in Table 1.

Non-neuroleptic medications have also been shown to be useful for reducing tic severity. These medications, however, have not been studied as extensively as neuroleptics. Non-neuroleptic medications with demonstrated efficacy in the treatment of TS include alpha-adrenergic agonists such as clonidine and guanfacine; neumuscular junction blocking agents such botulinum toxin; and centrally acting muscle relaxants such as baclofen. The most common side effects

Table 1. Neuroleptic drugs used in the treatment of tics.*

Medication	Starting dose (mg)	Usual dose range (mg/day)
Haloperidol	0.25–0.5	1–4
Pimozide	0.5–1	2–8
Risperidone	0.25–0.5	1.0–3.0
Fluphenazine	0.5–1.0	1.5–10
Ziprasidone	10–20	20–100

*Modified from Scahill *et al.*, 2006.

Table 2. Non-neuroleptic drugs used in the treatment of tics.*

Medication	Starting dose (mg)	Usual dose range (mg/day)
Clonidine	0.025–0.05	0.1–0.3
Guanfacine	0.5–1	1–3
Pergolide	0.025	0.1–0.4
Baclofen	10	40–60
Botulinum toxin	30–300 units into focal tic sites	

*Modified from Scahill *et al.*, 2006.

of non-neuroleptic medications, save botulinum toxin, is sedation. A list of non-neuroleptic medications commonly used for the treatment of tics is presented in Table 2.

Non-pharmacological treatment

Effective medications are also available to treat some of the neuro-psychological disorders commonly seen in patients with TS. The authors of several studies have determined that stimulant medications, such as methylphenidate and dextroamphetamine, can lessen ADHD symptoms in people with TS without worsening tic severity. The side effects of stimulant medications can be managed by initiating treatment slowly and reducing the dose as soon as side effects occur. A list of stimulant medications commonly used for the treatment of ADD and ADHD in patients with TS is presented in Table 3. For obsessive-compulsive symptoms that significiantly disrupt daily functioning, the serotonin reuptake inhibitors have been proven effective in some patients. A list of medications commonly used for the treatment of obsessive-compulsive symptoms in patients with TS is presented in Table 4.

Table 3. Stimulant medications for the treatment of ADD/ADHD in patients with TS.

Medication	Starting dose (mg)	Usual dose range (mg/kg/day)
Methylphenidate	0.3	0.3–1
Dextroamphetamine	2.5	5–20

Table 4. Medications used for the treatment of obsessive-compulsive symptoms in patients with TS.*

Medication	Starting dose (mg)	Usual dose range (mg/day)
Clomipramine	25–50	100–250
Fluoxetine	5–20	10–60
Sertraline	25–50	50–250
Fluvoxamine	25–50	50–350
Paroxetine	5–10	10–60

*Modified from Scahill *et al.*, 2006.

Psychotherapy has also been proven to provide benefit to patients with TS. Although pyschological problems do not cause TS, such problems may result from TS. Psychotherapy can help the person with TS better cope with the disorder and deal with the social and emotional problems that sometimes occur. More recently, specific behavioral treatments such as habit-reversal therapy, have emerged as promising modalities. The aim of these is to highten the patient's awareness of the tics and generate a competing response to the premonitory urge to have a tic. The advantage of a psychotherapeutic approach over drug treatment is the absence of medication side effects, lack of response to medication, and compliance with the medication regimen. Conversely, the disadvantages of psychotherapy is that it requires the active particpation of the patient, and the benefits are not immediate. These issues aside, psychotherapy may help build the child's functional behaviors and adaptive skills, as well as enhancing self-esteem.

Education

At school, children with TS may encounter social and educational challenges. Specifically, frequent tics, ADHD, learning disabilities, and obsessive-compulsive symptoms can greatly interfere with academic performance and social adjustment. For those reasons, modification of the school environment is not only a measure to stave off the effects of TS at school, it is actually the cornerstone of management. Children with TS should be placed in an educational setting that meets their individual needs. All students with TS need a tolerant and compassionate setting that both encourages them to work to their full potential and is flexible enough to accommodate their special needs. School accommodations can include small classrooms, private study rooms, tic breaks, untimed tests, test-taking in private rooms, and, for children with handwriting or other functional writing difficulties, scribes or tape recorders. Equally important is education of the child's teachers and peers. This can be accomplished through semiformal classroom presentations and educational videos on TS. Further information about school-based supports is available through the Tourette Syndrome Association of America (www.tsa-usa.org). The handbook "Teaching the Tiger" (www.hopepress.com) is available specifically for those involved in educating children with TS.

References

Albin RL, Mink JW. Recent advances in Tourette syndrome research. *Trends Neurosci.* 2006.29:423–428.

Cook CR, Blacher J. Evidence-based psychosocial treatments for tic disorders. *Clin Psychol Sci Prac.* 2007.14:252–267.

Scahill L, *et al.* Contemporary assessment and pharmacotherapy of Tourette syndrome. *NeuroRx.* 2006.3:192–206.

Tourette Syndrome. NIH publication No. 05-2163.

Tourette Syndrome Association of America: www.tsa-usa.org.

Zinner SH. Tourette syndrome — much more than tics. *Contemporary Pediatrics.* 2004.21:22–49.

INDEX